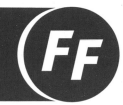

FAST FACTS

Indispensable Guides to Clinical Practice

Infant Nutrition

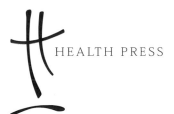

Alan Lucas
Medical Research Council Professor
University College Professor of Paediatric Nutrition
Director of the Childhood Nutrition Centre
Great Ormond Street Hospital for Children
and Institute of Child Health, London, UK

Stanley Zlotkin
Professor, Departments of Pediatrics and Nutritional
Sciences, and Research Fellow, Center for International
Health, University of Toronto;
Senior Scientist, Program in Metabolism
Research Institute, Hospital for Sick Children;
Head, Division of Gastroenterology and Nutrition
Hospital for Sick Children
Toronto, Ontario, Canada

HEALTH PRESS

Oxford

Fast Facts – Infant Nutrition
First published September 2003

Health Press Limited, Elizabeth House, Queen Street, Abingdon, Oxford
OX14 3JR, UK
Tel: +44 (0)1235 523233
Fax: +44 (0)1235 523238

Book orders can be placed by telephone or via the website.
For regional distributors or to order via the website, please go to:
www.fastfacts.com
For telephone orders, please call 01752 202301 (UK) or
1 800 538 1287 (North America, toll free).

Fast Facts is a trademark of Health Press Limited.

A CIP catalogue record for this title is available from the British Library.

ISBN 1-899541-93-4

Lucas, A (Alan)
Fast Facts – Infant Nutrition/
Alan Lucas, Stanley Zlotkin

Typeset by Zed, Oxford, UK.
Printed by Fine Print (Services) Ltd, Oxford, UK.

Printed with vegetable inks on fully biodegradable and
recyclable paper manufactured from sustainable forests.

444   001
Low emissions
during production

Low
chlorine

Sustainable
forests

Glossary of abbreviations

AA: arachidonic acid

AI: adequate intake

BMI: body mass index

BMR: basal metabolic rate

COMA: UK Committee on Medical Aspects

DHA: docosahexaenoic acid

GERD: gastroesophageal reflux disease

IDDM: insulin-dependent diabetes mellitus

LCPUFA: long-chain polyunsaturated fatty acid

NCHS: US National Center for Health Statistics

OES: oral electrolyte solution

ORT: oral rehydration therapy

PCB: polychlorinated biphenyl

PCDD: polychlorinated dibenzo-*p*-dioxin

PCDF: polychlorinated dibenzo-furan

RAE: retinol activity equivalent

RAST: radioallergosorbent test

RDA: recommended dietary allowance

SIDS: sudden infant death syndrome

WHO: World Health Organization

Introduction

Nutrition is the oldest branch of pediatrics and fundamental to it. Intensive research spans 200 years (Figure 1). Yet, paradoxically, nutrition has never developed as a formal specialty. Although virtually every parent seeks nutritional advice, and many hospitalized infants and children pose serious nutritional management problems, training of health professionals is minimal. This is likely to change in the light of recent advances in three areas that underpin a new understanding of the importance of early nutrition, namely:
- impact on long-term health and development
- effect on disease course
- health and safety aspects of early nutrition.

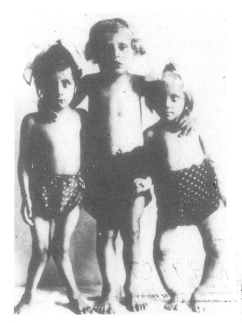

Figure 1 Nutrition has a long history. By the beginning of the last century, there was already a broad understanding of nutritional biochemistry and physiology, and of nutrient requirements. Funk coined the term 'vitamines' in 1911, and there has been long-standing interest in the treatment and prevention of specific nutrient deficiencies, such as rickets, depicted here.

The concept that internal or environmental stimuli, operating during critical periods of early development, can have lifelong effects on the organism has been termed 'programming'. Numerous animal studies support the idea that early nutrition can operate in this way. Brief early dietary manipulations have been shown to affect, into adulthood, brain development and propensity to disease, including diabetes, obesity, atherosclerosis and hypertension. Increasing evidence for these effects in humans has vastly raised the public health and clinical profile of pediatric nutrition.

Nutritional care may influence disease prognosis, clinical course, hospital stay, need for expensive treatments and requirement for healthcare resources in an increasing number of clinical circumstances, such as prematurity, gut disease, kidney disease and surgery. In sick infants, simple nutritional choices can influence the development of life-threatening disease processes, such as sepsis or necrotizing enterocolitis. Food given to infants can also have significant safety implications, some of which are discussed in this book.

Because early nutrition is important for the health and development of infants, it is critical that a broad range of health professionals involved in pediatrics gain insight into this emerging field. *Fast Facts – Infant Nutrition* provides practical, evidence-based guidance.

Significant postnatal adaptations are required to equip the infant for the major changes in nutrition and mode of feeding that occur after birth. These adaptions are:

- **mechanical** – neuromotor development permits coordinated sucking, swallowing and, later, mastication of foods
- **physiological** – notably changes in motor, digestive and absorptive functions of the gut and in other organs (liver, pancreas, kidneys) that equip the infant for postnatal feeding
- **biochemical** – changes in enzyme activity and biochemical pathways; for example the need to synthesize glucose endogenously (gluconeogenesis) after the transplacental supply of glucose from the mother suddenly ceases at birth
- **protective** – particularly developments in immune function and the mucosal barrier of the gut that occur as food-related exposure to potentially pathogenic organisms and antigens occurs postnatally.

Some of these postnatal adaptations are immediate (for instance gluconeogenesis); others develop gradually as the infant progresses from milk feeds towards a more adult diet; and some responses to early nutrition, which may be 'adaptive', are not manifest until later in life (the concept of 'programming'; see the chapter on Future trends).

In this chapter, selected physiological aspects relevant to practice are discussed.

Transition from fetal life

In utero, the fetus is mainly fed 'intravenously' via the placenta. However, at full term, the fetus also swallows approximately 500 mL of amniotic fluid daily, which provides approximately 25% of its protein requirement and a similar fluid intake to that of a breastfed baby. This 'enteral' feeding prenatally may help prepare the gut for feeding after birth. Postnatal feeding triggers further adaptive changes in the structure and function of the gut, and in metabolism, which equip the baby for milk feeding. If an infant, such as a sick intravenously fed baby, is deprived of enteral feeding after birth, the stimulus of food in the gut is removed and atrophic changes may occur in the intestine that impair its function and defense mechanisms. For this reason, 'minimal enteral feeding' is often used in sick babies who cannot be fully enterally fed, to maintain a stimulus for gut development.

Evolution of feeding skills

Some reflexes, notably those involving the cranial nerves, show a predictable pattern of maturation and extinction during early infancy and are necessary for normal early feeding patterns (Table 1.1). At 6 months, a baby has increasing control over its lips and tongue, and chewing movements begin. In addition, control of the neck and back muscles enables the infant to sit erect with support. Around 7–8 months, fine motor ability

TABLE 1.1

Infantile oral motor reflexes present from birth

Reflex	Description	Age at extinction
Rooting	Stroking around mouth elicits movement of head towards source of stimulus and latching onto nipple	3–4 months
Suck/ swallow	Stroking anterior third of tongue or center of lips elicits suck/swallow movements	6 months (evolution to mature sucking)
Biting	Stroking gum elicits rhythmic vertical biting motion of the jaw	6 months
Gag	Stimulus to the posterior three-quarters of the tongue and pharyngeal wall elicits constriction and elevation of the pharynx	Sensitivity shifts back to one-quarter of the tongue and the pharyngeal wall by adulthood
Extrusion	Food placed on the back of the tongue using a spoon is transferred to the front and expelled from the mouth	3–4 months

improves, allowing food to be grasped. A 1-year-old infant can usually sit without support, has good head control and can finger-feed.

Development of teeth

Teeth develop in utero, but normally do not begin to erupt through the gums until 6 months after birth. By 12 months, 4–8 primary teeth have usually erupted, and then the remainder appear during the second year. The incisors allow food to be cut and appear first, and by 1 year molars are present to grind food (Figure 1.1). Exceptions to the sequence of eruption are uncommon. Late eruption is rarely significant but has been associated with hypothyroidism and rickets.

Digestion and absorption

In infants, digestion and absorption of most breast-milk nutrients is as efficient as in adults. For example, the key enzymes for disaccharide

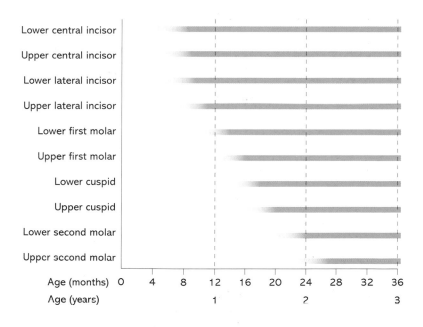

Figure 1.1 The order of eruption of deciduous teeth. The paler areas represent the normal variation in age at tooth eruption.

digestion approach adult levels by birth (Figure 1.2). Such physiological maturation of the infant's intestine is relevant to the infant's readiness for weaning (see Chapter 7, page 57). In contrast, the bioavailability of nutrients such as zinc, iron and saturated fats from other foods like unmodified cows' milk (which is now considered inappropriate for young infants) is reduced.

Fat absorption is less efficient at birth than at 6 months. Nevertheless, even in newborns, 85–90% of the fat in breast milk is absorbed, whereas 'butterfat' from cows' milk is relatively poorly absorbed in early infancy. Blends of vegetable oils are now used in infant formulas. Those with high palmitate levels result in reduced saturated fat (and calcium) absorption (see Chapter 4, page 35), though oil blends can be devised from which fat absorption approximates that from breast milk.

The infant's digestive capacity must be taken into account when choosing age-appropriate foods. For example, starch digestion is limited at birth owing to low pancreatic amylase secretion.

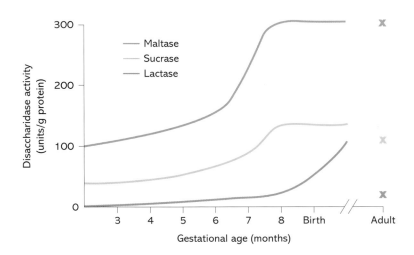

Figure 1.2 Development of disaccharidase activity in the jejunal mucosa of the human fetus. Adapted from: Johnson TR, Moore WM, Jeffries JE, eds. *Children are Different – Developmental Physiology*. 2nd edn. Columbus: Ross Labs, 1987.

Renal development

At birth, glomerular filtration rate (GFR) is only approximately 30% of adult values and remains below adult levels until around the third year (Figure 1.3). The low GFR of the neonatal kidney limits its capacity to excrete the end-products of protein metabolism, such as urea, or excess solutes, such as sodium, potassium and chloride. Though nutrient requirements for growth are large, less than 50% of the solute ingested from appropriate nutritional sources is utilized. Any excess beyond requirements, called the renal solute load, must be excreted. The amount of water required for renal excretion is determined mainly by the size of the renal solute load, which depends on diet. Under normal environmental conditions, renal solute load is low in relation to the amount of water available, and so water balance is not threatened. Under adverse conditions, however, water requirements for excretion may exceed availability, resulting in tissue dehydration, retention of potentially toxic products and renal failure (Table 1.2). Infant foods must, therefore, yield sufficiently low renal solute loads to provide a safety margin in the event of fluid imbalance. Human breast milk and modern adapted infant formulas allow such a margin. Unmodified

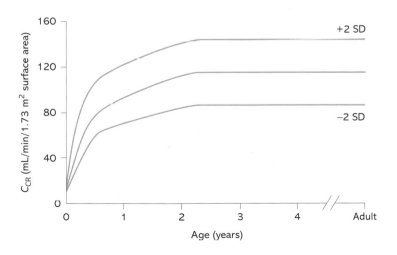

Figure 1.3 Changes in glomerular filtration rate with age. C_{CR}, creatinine clearance; SD, standard deviation.

TABLE 1.2

Factors affecting fluid balance

Increased water loss
- Diarrhea/vomiting
- Fever
- High environmental temperature

Restricted fluid intake
- Vomiting
- Concentrated infant formulas

Impaired renal concentrating ability
- Primary or secondary renal disease

cows' milk, however, with its high protein and electrolyte content, does not, and in conditions that reduce water availability, such as diarrhea, potentially dangerous hyperosmolarity can develop.

Immunological development

A newborn infant has circulating antibodies (mainly immunoglobulin G, IgG) that were acquired prenatally from its mother via the placenta. In addition, breast milk provides the immunologically immature infant passive immunity in the form of immunoglobulin A (IgA) in the gut lumen, which helps protect the infant from infection via the gastrointestinal and upper respiratory tracts. The protective mechanisms in operation in the infant gut are shown in Table 1.3.

An important adaptation of the gut to extrauterine life is the development of a mucosal barrier. This overlies the microvillous surface and protects against penetration by antigens present in the intestinal lumen. A newborn infant must deal with bacterial colonization of the gut, viruses, endo- and enterotoxins produced by bacteria and food (mainly milk) antigens. Protection against mucosal invasion includes both local (IgA) and systemic responses and, in breastfed infants, milk IgA and other antimicrobial factors (see Chapter 4, page 35). If

TABLE 1.3

Protective mechanisms in the infant gut

Intraluminal

- Gastric barrier
- Proteolysis
- Peristalsis
- Antimicrobial factors in breast milk

Mucosal surface

- Mucosal coat
- Microvillous membrane

Immunological

- Secretory immunoglobulin A system

potentially immunologically active substances penetrate the mucosal barrier they can cause inflammatory and allergic reactions, which may result in diarrhea (including bloody stools), eczema (itchy dermatitis, particularly on the flexor surfaces) and wheezing or respiratory distress.

Nutritional 'programming'

Increasing evidence shows early nutrition has major so-called 'programming' effects on long-term health, including effects on cognitive function, bone health, and cardiovascular disease and its risk factors. Thus early nutrition may be an important environmental influence on long-term cell-biological and physiological development of the organism. These aspects are discussed in the final chapter.

Traditionally, calculation of nutrient and energy requirements in the first 6 months for infants born at term has been based on the average composition of breast milk (Table 2.1). The precise dietary intake of breastfed babies is, however, unknown and there is also uncertainty about the ideal growth pattern during infancy. Indeed, in the West, there have recently been marked changes in infant growth patterns, perhaps related to the changing eating habits of families. Animal and human data indicate that early diet may have long-term consequences for future growth, development and morbidity. However, optimal nutrient intakes for infants have not been assessed in these terms, and so appropriate dietary goals continue to be disputed.

Various terms have been used to attempt to define nutrient intakes or needs, for instance recommended dietary allowances (RDAs). The population guidelines for infants are now often not referred to as RDAs because there is less certainty about the exact nutrient needs of individual infants at this age. The new term used to describe recommended nutrient intakes for infants is the estimated adequate intake (AI). For infants, the AI is the mean intake of individual nutrients in an adequate volume of human milk, or, for older infants, a combination of milk and weaning foods. Both the AI and the RDA are to be used as a goal for individual nutrient intake. The values are intended to cover the needs of nearly all healthy infants in the first 12 months of life (Table 2.2).

Energy

Total dietary energy is the sum of the energy contents of carbohydrate, fat and protein. About 50% of the energy intake of a healthy breast-fed infant is fat (Table 2.3). Reducing fat intake in infancy and applying the principles of healthy eating appropriate for adults is inadvisable and may result in insufficient available energy (see Chapter 7, page 57).

The energy a baby obtains from its food is either stored (deposited) in new tissue during growth or in body fat, or expended (burnt off) to

TABLE 2.1

Composition of human breast milk

Component	Human milk
Energy	680 kcal/liter
Protein	10 g/liter
Whey	72%
Casein	28%
Fat	39 g/liter
Medium-chain triglyceride	2%
Long-chain triglyceride	98%
Carbohydrate*	72 g/liter
Lactose	100%
Minerals	
Calcium	280 mg/liter
Phosphorus	140 mg/liter
Magnesium	35 mg/liter
Sodium	180 mg/liter
Potassium	525 mg/liter
Chloride	420 mg/liter
Zinc	1200 µg/liter
Copper	250 µg/liter
Iron	300 µg/liter
Fat-soluble vitamins	
Vitamin A	2230 IU/liter
Vitamin D	22 IU/liter
Vitamin E	2.3 IU/liter
Vitamin K	2.1 µg/liter
Water-soluble vitamins	
Thiamin/vitamin B_1	210 µg/liter
Riboflavin/vitamin B_2	350 µg/liter
Pyridoxine/vitamin B_6	93 µg/liter
Niacin	1.5 mg/liter
Biotin	4 µg/liter
Pantothenic acid	1.8 mg/liter
Folic acid	85 µg/liter
Vitamin B_{12}	1 µg/liter
Vitamin C	40 mg/liter

*In addition, human milk contains oligosaccharides, nucleotides and long-chain polyunsaturated fatty acids (see Chapter 5, page 46)

TABLE 2.2

Estimated adequate intake for major nutrients in infants (Dietary Reference Intakes USA/Canada 2000)

	Age (months)	
	0–6	6–12
Protein (g)	13	14
Fat-soluble vitamins		
A (µg retinol activity equivalents, RAE)	400	500
D (µg)	5	5
E (µg)	4	6
K (µg)	2	2.5
Water-soluble vitamins		
C (mg)	40	50
Thiamin (mg)	0.2	0.3
Riboflavin (mg)	0.3	0.4
Niacin (mg)	2	6
B_6 (mg)	0.1	0.3
Folate (µg)	65	80
B_{12} (µg)	0.4	0.5
Minerals		
Calcium (mg)	210	270
Phosphorus (mg)	100	275
Magnesium (mg)	30	75
Iron (mg)	0.27	11
Zinc (mg)	2	3
Iodine (µg)	110	130

TABLE 2.3

Energy and macronutrient distribution in typical mature breast milk

Nutrient	Amount (g/100 mL)	Energy (kcal/100 mL)	Proportion of total energy in diet (%)
Protein	1	4	6
Carbohydrate	7	28	41
Fat	4	36	53
Total		**68**	**100**

support the basal metabolic rate, the energy cost of activity and the cost of maintaining body temperature (thermogenesis). Energy requirements for growth in later infancy are much smaller than usually assumed. By the age of 9 months, the energy cost of an infant's growth has fallen to less than 10% of intake, whereas the cost of activity is approximately 40%. Much of the energy cost of activity is 'involuntary' (e.g. spontaneous movements, crying) and may be influenced by the infant's temperament. The amount of energy needed and the percentage of the total requirement for each component is shown in Figure 2.1 and Table 2.4.

Proteins and amino acids

In infants, protein intake per kilogram body weight is greater than for adults. In mammals, the nutrient factor that has the greatest correlation with postnatal growth rate is milk protein.

The essential amino acids in human nutrition are arginine, lysine, leucine, isoleucine, valine, methionine, phenylalanine, threonine and tryptophan. Because of late development of certain enzymes of amino-

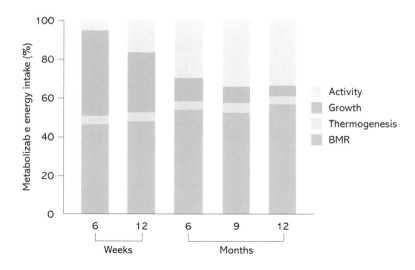

Figure 2.1 Components of energy expenditure as a percentage of energy intake during infancy. BMR, basal metabolic rate.

TABLE 2.4

Energy needs in infancy (kcal/day)

	Age				
	6 weeks	12 weeks	6 months	9 months	12 months
Energy cost of growth	199	176	71	66	47
Basic metabolic rate	206	266	343	395	450
Energy cost of activity	26	93	201	270	274
Thermogenesis	23	28	32	38	40
Total energy intake	**454**	**563**	**647**	**769**	**811**

acid metabolism, the newborn infant may have a temporarily increased requirement for cysteine and histidine, and perhaps taurine (which is now included in infant formulas).

The two main classes of milk protein are whey and casein. Human milk generally has a higher proportion of whey (on average 60% of total protein – range 43–89%), while cows' milk has a higher proportion of casein (only 20% whey). In human whey, α-lactalbumin is the dominant protein, followed by lactoferrin. In contrast, the major whey protein in cows' milk is β-lactoglobulin, which is absent from human milk and potentially antigenic when fed to human infants.

During lactation, milk protein content falls substantially from more than 20 g to approximately 10 g/liter, possibly reflecting an adaptation to the infant's decreasing protein requirement with advancing age.

Practice point: supplementation

- For poorly growing babies, clinicians often incorrectly assume that energy supplementation is all that is required. In fact, a broad range of nutrients, and in particular protein, is needed to promote growth.

Fat

The fat content of milk from different mothers is variable, and also changes throughout lactation, diurnally and between breasts. However, the major variation is during an individual feed – fat rises from an average 2 g/100 mL in foremilk to 4 g/100 mL in hindmilk. The nutritional quality of milk mechanically or manually expressed from the breast, therefore, will depend on whether it is foremilk, hindmilk or a combination.

Cows' milk and human milk have a similar fat content (98% triglyceride); the principal difference is the fatty acid pattern. Breast-milk fatty acids are markedly influenced by maternal diet. Vegetarians, for instance, consume more long-chain fatty acids than those on a mixed diet. Human milk generally has a higher proportion of unsaturated fatty acids than cows' milk and a greater concentration of the essential fatty acids (see below).

Breast-milk lipids are in complex membrane-covered globules that, unsurprisingly, cannot be mimicked in infant formula. Most modern formulas contain a mixture of vegetable oils, adjusted to mimic the pattern of fatty acid saturation and chain-lengths found in breast milk. However, the positioning of the three fatty acids on the glycerol backbone (to constitute a triglyceride) is quite different in human milk and vegetable fats, with potentially important implications for infants (see Chapter 5, page 46).

Essential fatty acids and long-chain polyunsaturated fatty acids.

Linoleic and α-linolenic acids are essential (precursor) dietary fatty acids that are required for brain development and prostaglandin synthesis. Frank essential fatty acid deficiency, which is associated with skin lesions and retarded growth, is unusual.

Two groups of long-chain polyunsaturated fatty acids (LCPUFAs), with greater than 18-carbon chain length, are the subjects of growing interest. They are derived from linoleic acid (one example is arachidonic acid, AA) and from α-linolenic acid (for example docosahexaenoic acid, DHA). LCPUFAs are synthesized from precursor fatty acids. They are found in high concentrations in cell-membrane phospholipids, notably in the central nervous system and retina, and are important for normal neurological function. In addition, LCPUFAs are precursors for eicosanoids, which are important modulators and mediators of many essential biological processes.

Rapid accumulation of LCPUFAs in the brain, particularly DHA, occurs between the third trimester and 18 months postpartum. Human milk contains both parent precursor fatty acids *and* LCPUFAs. However, infant formulas have traditionally contained only the parent essential fatty acids. Whether infants can adequately synthesize LCPUFAs from these is discussed in Chapter 5 (page 46).

TABLE 2.5

Effects of mineral deficiency

Mineral	Deficiency
Calcium	Tetany, bone demineralization, arrhythmias, paralytic ileus, fits
Phosphorus	Phosphate deficiency syndrome may arise, particularly in infants fed by total parenteral nutrition: listlessness, poor feeding, rapid shallow breathing, muscle weakness, impaired oxygen release from hemoglobin, bone disease, nephrocalcinosis
Magnesium	Weakness, poor feeding, failure to thrive, paralytic ileus, calcium-resistant tetany, fits, apnea
Iodine	Endemic goiter in areas where human milk is deficient; soy formulas would have low iodine if not supplemented
Iron	Depressed cognitive and motor development, increased fearfulness, wariness and fatigue, less exploration of the environment
Zinc	Acrodermatitis syndrome – there may be delayed diagnosis if signs are mistaken for 'nappy rash' of another etiology. It may also be inherited as a rare autosomal recessive disorder. Also mild deficiency in infancy, or later, may be associated with reduced growth, loss of appetite, impaired taste acuity and perhaps pica. Impaired immune responses, poor wound healing

Carbohydrate

Lactose is the dominant and unique carbohydrate in mammalian milk. It enhances calcium absorption, promotes the growth of nonpathogenic lactobacilli and may help to create a favorable gut flora that protects against gastroenteritis. Most infant formulas provide lactose as the sole or predominant carbohydrate source, though human infants may effectively digest other carbohydrates, such as sucrose, amylose and maltodextrins, incorporated into some formulas (see Figure 1.2).

Sodium

Two factors influence dietary recommendations for sodium: first, the concern that high salt intake might result in dangerous hypernatremia in conditions in which excessive water is lost, such as diarrhea; second, the theoretical, though unconvincing, evidence that early salt intake might predispose to high blood pressure later in life.

Minerals and vitamins

The effects of mineral or vitamin deficiency or excess are summarized in Tables 2.5 and 2.6 (over page); selected nutrients are also discussed in later chapters.

TABLE 2.6

Effects of vitamin deficiency or excess

Vitamin	Deficiency	Excess
Vitamin A	Xerophthalmia, susceptibility to infection, keratinization of mucous membranes, blindness	Raised intracranial pressure, dry skin, loss of hair, brittle bones, irritability
Thiamine (B_1)	Anorexia, irritability, fatigue, edema, heart failure, constipation, peripheral neuropathy	
Riboflavin (B_2)	Cheilosis, angular stomatitis, impaired fatty acid oxidation, iron metabolism	
Niacin	Diarrhea, dermatitis, neurological disturbance	
Pyridoxine (B_6)	Convulsions, dermatitis, weakness, anemia	
Vitamin B_{12}	Pernicious anemia, central nervous system damage	
Folic acid	Megaloblastic anemia, retarded growth, gastrointestinal disturbance	
Pantothenic acid	No dietary deficiency state described in man	
Biotin	Possibly skin rashes	
Vitamin C	Biochemical deficiency may arise in newborn period, overt scurvy rare < 3 months of age	
Vitamin D	Rickets, tetany Maternal deficiency may rarely result in neonatal rickets The very small amount in breast milk is occasionally insufficient, especially if light exposure is minimal	Hypercalcemia, ectopic calcification, failure to thrive
Vitamin E	Clinical disease states poorly defined, reduces postnatal red cell hemolysis	
Vitamin K	Hemorrhagic disease of the newborn	Excess of water-soluble analog can cause hemolytic anemia

Growth is a critical biological attribute that distinguishes the pediatric population. It is the traditional test of overall nutritional status and is deranged in many conditions. Proper assessment of growth can have major biological, clinical, public health and social value, but health professionals are frequently inadequately trained in the collection, processing and interpretation of growth data.

Measurement of growth

The standard body measurements used in practice are weight, length and head circumference (Table 3.1 and Figure 3.1). In healthy infants, body weight is a 'summary' of many aspects of growth and, given appropriate equipment, it is the simplest and most accurate measurement. More sophisticated scales reduce infant movement artefacts by damping or automatically averaging several weights. Length measurement is more difficult and requires training; inaccurate measurements have little value.

Measurement of length and weight allows indices of weight for length, such as body mass index (BMI), to be calculated. Other body measurements, such as mid-arm and other circumferences and skin-fold thicknesses, are generally not clinically useful in infancy.

Growth charts

Growth is most commonly assessed using growth charts that are based on sizes of babies measured at different ages, though not necessarily the same babies at each age. At each time point, a family of centiles is derived for weight, length and head circumference. Thus the 25th, 50th and 75th centiles define the value, say for body weight, below which 25%, 50% and 75% of the population lie, respectively. With secular changes in infant feeding practices, the growth of babies has changed over time, and modern babies no longer grow according to charts devised 30–40 years ago. In many countries growth charts are being updated. The most modern charts used routinely in the UK, and

TABLE 3.1

Taking growth measurements

Weight

- An infant or toddler should always be weighed naked on a self-zeroing or regularly calibrated scale

Head circumference

- Head circumference should be measured midway between the eyebrows and the hairline at the front of the head and the occipital prominence at the back (Figure 3.1). Appropriate thin plastic, metal or disposable paper tape should be used; sewing tape is not recommended for this purpose

Supine length

- Infants (and children up to approximately 18 months) should be measured in the supine position (on their back) by two people with equipment comprising both a headboard and moveable footboard (Figure 3.1). While one person holds the head against the headboard, with the head facing upwards in the Frankfort plane (an imaginary line from the center of the ear hole to the lower border of the eye socket), a second person measures the length by bringing the footboard up to the heels. Downward pressure is applied to the child's knees to ensure that the legs are flat (this does not carry any risk of hip dislocation)

illustrated here, are derived from the growth of modern infants. These charts are based on nine centiles (0.4th, 2nd, 9th, 25th, 50th, 75th, 90th, 98th and 99.6th), with each centile position mathematically 'smoothed' across the age range to produce a tidy chart (Figure 3.2).

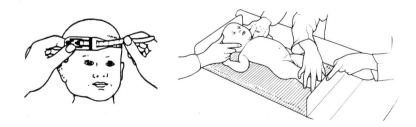

Figure 3.1 Measurement of head circumference and length. Reproduced by permission of the Child Growth Foundation, London, UK.

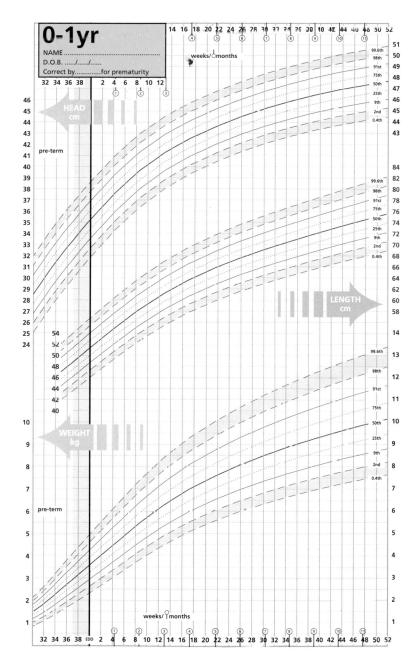

Figure 3.2 Infant growth chart for boys' head circumference, supine length and weight. Reproduced by permission of the Child Growth Foundation, London, UK.

These centiles were chosen because they are two-thirds of a standard deviation apart. Thus, the 2nd and 98th centiles, which are commonly used in many areas of medicine to define the 'normal' range, are two standard deviations either side of the mean. Nine-centile charts, however, provide a further pair of more deviant centiles (0.4th and 99.6th) to define a smaller, more extreme population that can be practically referred for growth problems.

It is important to note that such charts do not describe the growth of any individual baby, and centile-crossing frequently occurs in infancy. There are a number of reasons for this (Table 3.2), and healthcare professionals must distinguish acceptable from suspect variation in centile position (see below).

Use of growth charts. The principal clinical purpose of using growth charts is to identify disorders of growth, either related directly to nutrition or various disease processes or indirectly to social factors, such as neglect and deprivation. Growth charts may be used in different ways, and recently developed approaches can be helpful (see below).

TABLE 3.2

Reasons for variation in centile position on growth charts in normal infants

- Birth size largely reflects maternal size. Centile-crossing occurs as the baby's genetic growth potential is revealed, with stabilization occurring in the second year

- Large babies tend to cross centiles downwards and small babies upwards (tendency to regress to the mean)

- Growth does not occur smoothly but in spurts, producing short-term variability

- If weight measurements are made very close together, spurious variability can arise because underlying weight gain (only 6 g/day in late infancy) is masked by timing of bladder or rectal emptying and feeds (a single milk feed may weigh > 200 g)

- Inaccurate measurement is a major cause of spuriously erratic growth, particularly in length, which requires training to measure

Single measurements may be used to screen populations for potential problems requiring investigation. For example, measurement of head circumference at birth is a useful screening test for developmental problems of the brain, such as microcephaly or hydrocephalus. A body measurement at any age that falls below the 0.4th or above the 99.6th centile warrants investigation, referral or at least explanation.

Sequential measurements. Sequential body weight measurements may show downward (or upward) centile-crossing that is cause for concern. Failure to grow adequately in infancy is termed 'failure to thrive'. Given the variety of reasons for variation in centile position in healthy infants, recent efforts have been made to make 'failure to thrive' a formal rather than an arbitrary diagnosis. New, special acetate overlays allow the investigator to determine whether an infant at any starting point on a chart proceeds to grow better or worse than, say, the slowest growing 5% of a population of infants (Figure 3.3).

Undernutrition initially affects body-weight gain and, if chronic, retards linear growth and eventually, and most significantly, brain growth (head circumference). Thus, acute undernutrition will result in reduced weight for length (wasting), and chronic undernutrition in reduced height for age (stunting). With the use of specialized charts, assessment of weight for length need not be arbitrary. Figure 3.4 shows centile distributions of BMI, calculated as weight (kilograms) divided by length (meters) squared. These charts are not reliable in early infancy, but a 1-year-old child with a BMI of 13 would be unusually thin (less than the 0.4th centile), whereas one with a BMI of 22 would have unusual excess body weight for length (BMI greater than 99.6th centile).

Routine measurement of growth

While parents and some health professionals might regard routine growth monitoring in infancy as a matter of obvious importance, each aspect needs careful appraisal. Overfrequent monitoring or uncritical data interpretation can lead to increased parental anxiety, unnecessary referral, inappropriate medical management or even unjustified childcare proceedings. The acid test of the value of any screening program is that it leads to intervention of proven value.

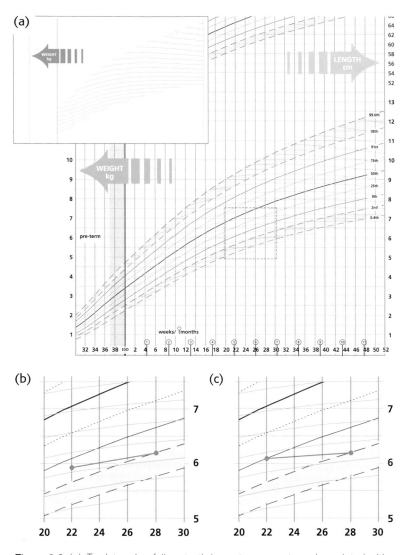

Figure 3.3 (a) To determine failure to thrive, a transparent overlay printed with thrive lines (here shown in green, inset and superimposed) is placed over a growth chart (see Figure 3.2). In this case, a chart for girls' weights is illustrated. The child's weight is measured at two points a minimum of 1 month apart and plotted on the chart. The slope of the line (blue) joining the points should be greater than that of the nearest thrive line. Thus the examples show (b) a child whose growth is adequate and (c) a child whose growth gives cause for concern. Reproduced by permission of the Child Growth Foundation, London, UK.

Monitoring body weight is potentially valuable when screening for 'failure to thrive'. Most children with organic causes of failure to thrive have associated features. Suboptimal nutrition probably accounts for most cases of 'isolated' failure to thrive, which is often undiagnosed

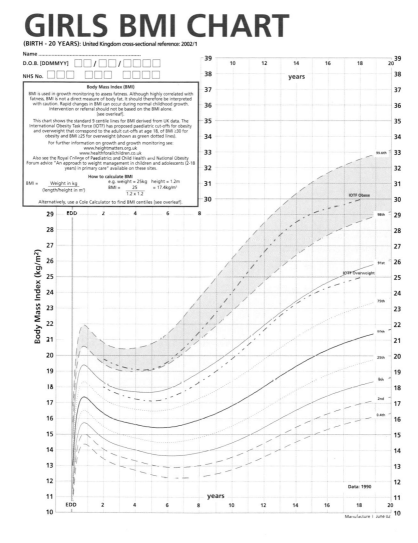

GIRLS BMI CHART

(BIRTH - 20 YEARS): United Kingdom cross-sectional reference: 2002/1

Figure 3.4 Body mass index chart for girls from birth to adulthood. Reproduced by permission of the Child Growth Foundation, London, UK.

and self-limiting and often occurs in unexceptional circumstances. The question whether intervention in such cases is clinically valuable, in terms of long-term health and development, is under-researched, but it seems prudent to identify failure to thrive by routine screening, exclude organic causes and attempt to improve nutritional status. At a minimum, babies should be weighed at birth, at the time of immunization and at an 8- or 9-month check. However, frequent weight monitoring, for example weekly or fortnightly, is pointless and likely to yield confusing results (see Table 3.2).

Birth length is not predictive of later length. Measurement of stature in the first year of life has uncertain value. Screening of body length or height for growth hormone deficiency or Turner's syndrome would normally be done beyond infancy. Nevertheless, while infant length measurement has limited value for assessing stature, up to four measurements in infancy can be justified for assessing the relationship between weight and length in screening for failure to thrive or undernutrition (see above). But health professionals need training in length measurement (see Table 3.1 and Figure 3.1).

Detailed growth monitoring of children with clinical problems affecting nutrition and growth is valuable diagnostically, for guiding intervention and monitoring progress.

What to do when growth is faltering

Preliminary assessment. The role of the health practitioner is to determine why growth is faltering and, if possible, initiate corrective intervention. The initial step is a preliminary baseline or screening assessment of nutritional status. This process is similar to that used in the initial assessment of a patient's general medical status, based on history and examination.

History. It is important to ask questions about:
- past health
- previous hospitalizations or operations, which may have resulted in poor food intake
- feeding behavior
- any emesis and stool pattern, to assess likelihood of excess nutrient losses.

When assessing nutrient intake in infants, the most important single aspect is to ensure adequate milk intake (breast milk or formula) for age since this is the major component of an infant's diet (Table 3.3). After 4–6 months, breast milk alone is unlikely to meet requirements for protein and other nutrients, and the infant may become deficient in vitamins A and D and iron, and may show a reduced growth rate. In the USA, iron deficiency may arise if low-iron formulas (unavailable in Europe) are used over a prolonged period. Significant deviations from the typical pattern of intake (Table 3.3) may provide a pointer to inadequate nutrition as a cause of faltering growth.

Examination should include simple physical inspection of the child for obvious wasting, and collection of growth data, notably weight and length assessed using standard charts. Such examination will categorize the child as 'normal' or, if any of the following features are present, as needing further assessment:
- normal growth patterns not being followed
- inadequate food intake or inappropriate food choice
- excessive nutrient losses
- retarded feeding development.

Detailed nutritional assessment. The purpose of the assessment is to determine whether nutrient deficiencies are present; if so, to identify possible causes; and to help direct nutritional therapy. The assessment should include:
- a more detailed history
- assessment of food intake and eating behavior
- physical examination for signs of nutrient deficiencies, such as decreased adipose tissue and pale conjunctiva
- anthropometry, perhaps including the use of specialized charts, to assess failure to thrive and BMI
- specific diagnostic investigations linked to the outcome of the history, dietary assessment and anthropometry.

For example, in a child with a history of excessive unmodified cows' milk intake at a young age, with pale conjunctiva, a hemoglobin count and serum ferritin concentration should be obtained to rule out iron-deficiency anemia. Whenever poor intake adequately explains growth

TABLE 3.3

Typical guidelines for food intake of infants

	4–6 months
Milk	*Minimum 600 mL breast or infant formula daily*
Dairy products and substitutes	• Cows' milk products can be used in weaning after 4 months (e.g. yoghurt, custard, cheese sauce)
Starchy foods	*Introduce after 4 months* • Mix smooth cereal with milk; use low-fiber cereals (e.g. rice-based) • Mash or purée starchy vegetables
Vegetables and fruits	*Introduce after 4 months* • Use soft-cooked vegetables and fruit as a smooth purée
Meat and meat alternatives	*Introduce after 4 months* • Use soft-cooked meat/pulses • Add no salt or sugar, or minimum quantities, to food during or after cooking
Occasional foods	• Choose low-sugar desserts; avoid high-salt foods

6–9 months	9–12 months
500–600 mL breast milk, infant formula or follow-on formula daily	*500–600 mL breast milk or infant milk daily*
• Also use any milk to mix solids • Hard cheese (e.g. Cheddar) can be cubed or grated and used as finger food	• Also use any milk to mix solids
2–3 servings daily • Start to introduce some wholemeal bread and cereals • Foods can be a more solid 'lumpier' texture • Begin to give finger foods (e.g. toast)	*3–4 servings daily* • Encourage wholemeal products; discourage foods with added sugar (biscuits, cakes, etc.) • Starchy foods can be of normal adult texture
2 servings daily • Raw soft fruit and vegetables (e.g. banana, melon, tomato) may be used as finger foods • Cooked vegetables and fruit can be a coarser, mashed texture	*3–4 servings daily* • Encourage lightly-cooked or raw foods • Chopped or finger food texture is unsuitable • Unsweetened orange juice with meals, especially if diet is meat free
1 serving daily • Soft-cooked minced or puréed meat/fish/pulses • Chopped hard-cooked egg can be used as a finger food	*Minimum 1 serving daily from animal source or 2 from vegetable sources* • In a vegetarian diet use a mixture of different vegetable and starchy foods (macaroni cheese, dhal, rice)
• Encourage savory foods rather than sweet ones • Fruit juices are not necessary – try to restrict to mealtimes or alternatively offer water/milk	• May use moderate amounts of butter, margarine. Small amounts of jam (if necessary) on bread • Try to limit salty foods (e.g. many processed foods)

failure, there is no need to pursue medical causes or look for nutrient losses unless the child fails to respond to adequate intake.

The most common cause of infant undernutrition is inadequate feeding, either inadvertent or intentional. However, a sizeable proportion of infants will have organic diagnoses that require specialist attention. These fall into three categories:

- those that cause decreased food ingestion, notably feeding dysfunction or dysphagia
- nutrient malabsorption – notably cystic fibrosis, but also a wide variety of gut disorders including enteropathies, short bowel syndrome and liver disease
- increased nutrient needs, for example in heart disease or chronic infection.

Breastfeeding is the physiological mode of feeding for human infants. Only in the last 70 years have substitutes for breast milk been used on a large scale.

Benefits to infants

Breastfeeding is recommended for all infants, with very few exceptions (see below). This section reviews the benefits to the infant as a basis for medical counseling of mothers.

Unique properties of human milk. A general argument in favor of breastfeeding is the unique, species-specific and complex biological nature of breast milk, which cannot be mimicked by formula manufacturers.

Nutritional aspects (see Table 2.1). Some classes of breast-milk nutrients – long-chain polyunsaturated fatty acids (prevalent components of the central nervous system), nucleotides (with widespread effects, notably on the immune system) and oligosaccharides (the third most prevalent nutrient category after fat and lactose) – have only recently been considered for inclusion in milk formulas. Attempts to mimic even the nutrient content of breast milk (let alone the non-nutrient content, see below) are prevented by its biological complexity (e.g. fats in breast milk are contained in globules covered in cell membrane, Figure 4.1). Many nutrient (and non-nutrient) factors in breast milk have never been put into infant formulas. Theoretically, the absence of these factors in the diet might disadvantage the infant. Nevertheless, the potential value of adding any such factor, even if feasible, into an infant formula now requires rigorous efficacy and safety testing.

Immunological and antimicrobial aspects. Human milk is a living tissue (Figure 4.2) containing live cells (immunocompetent lymphocytes and macrophages) and has numerous factors with potential antimicrobial activity (Table 4.1). The principal factor is the immunoglobulin secretory IgA that comprises a wide variety of

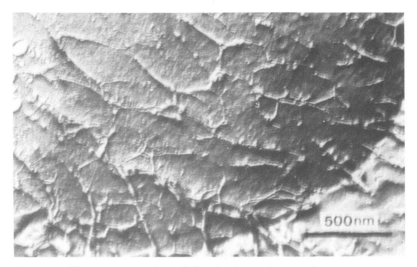

Figure 4.1 The appearance of a milk-fat globule on electron microscopy.

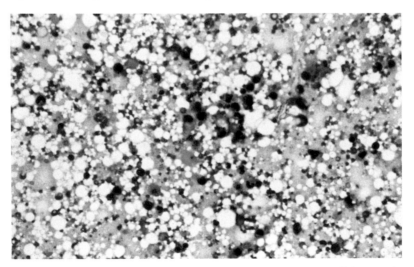

Figure 4.2 Histological appearance of human breast milk showing cellularity and milk-fat globules.

antibodies to viruses, bacteria and their toxins. The antibodies produced in milk are directed against organisms to which the mother has been exposed via the gut and the respiratory tract, and which her infant might be likely to meet in the same environment. Experimentally, the oral administration of non-pathogenic bacteria to lactating mothers

TABLE 4.1

Antimicrobial factors in breast milk*

Factor	Notes
Secretory IgA	Antibodies against a wide range of bacterial, viral, parasitic and fungal antigens
IgG and IgM	Low levels
Complement	Low levels
Lactoferrin	Binds iron, may deprive microorganisms of iron as a growth factor
Lysozyme	Lyses bacterial cell walls
Oligosaccharides and glycoconjugates	May bind with organisms
Nucleotides	May promote cell-mediated immunity
Antiviral factors	Including interferon

*Numerous other factors with potential antimicrobial roles have been identified, but IgA is likely to be the most important factor

results in type-specific IgA and IgA-secreting cells appearing in their milk within a few days. This has led to the hypothesis that there is a selective transfer ('homing') of sensitized lymphocytes from the gut to the breast, making the protection specific to the mother's own infant. The combined impact of antimicrobial factors (see Table 4.1) against infection is discussed below.

Possible 'messenger' substances in human milk. Breast milk contains numerous hormones and growth factors (Table 4.2). Animal and some human data suggest that these may be absorbed from the gut. Possibly, then, the lactating mother, in addition to providing nutrients and anti-infective factors, exerts some control over neonatal metabolism and development through the mediation of 'chemical messengers' and trophic factors secreted into her milk.

Enzymes. Breast milk contains several enzymes. A lipase in breast milk, activated by bile salts in the infant's gut, may play a significant part in the infant's fat digestion. Breast-milk amylase may compensate for the slow development of salivary amylase in infants.

Proposed health benefits. A general problem with all studies comparing breast- versus formula-fed infants is the potential confounding effect of demographic differences between these groups (e.g. education, socioeconomic status and positive health behavior). Nevertheless, observational studies collectively underpin current promotion of breastfeeding by numerous health organizations worldwide.

Reduced incidence of infection. Recent studies provide evidence that, even in developed countries, breastfeeding protects against gastrointestinal and respiratory infections and decreases the risk of otitis media. A UK study showed infants exclusively breastfed for 13 weeks or more had fewer gastrointestinal and respiratory illnesses during the first year compared with formula-fed infants (and were less likely to have had respiratory illness in 7 years of follow-up). Breastfed infants supplemented with formula or food before 4 months appear more likely to develop otitis media. A recent meta-analysis of risk factors for acute otitis media showed the risk decreased with breastfeeding for at least 3 months.

TABLE 4.2

Examples of hormones reported in breast milk

- Steroids
- Thyroxine
- Gonadotropins
- Luteinizing hormone-releasing hormone
- Thyrotropin-releasing hormone
- Thyroid-stimulating hormone
- Adrenocorticotropic hormone
- Prolactin
- Erythropoietin
- Melatonin
- Epidermal growth factor
- Prostaglandins
- Calcitonin

Protection against allergies. The incidence of atopic disease in
infants has been estimated at up to 10%, but may be closer to 2%. The
wide range of reported incidence is due to variable diagnostic criteria,
poor study designs and the high incidence of self-diagnosis. In the only
randomized trial of human milk versus formula milk (possible in
preterm infants who can be randomly assigned to donated banked
breast milk or formula), feeding human milk did not reduce clinical
atopy in infants with no genetic predisposition; however, in those with
a family history of atopy, feeding cows'-milk-based formula in the early
weeks greatly increased the risk of atopic disease (i.e. the combined
incidence of eczema, food and drug reactions and wheezing). Further
observational studies on full-term infants with a positive family history
of atopy (in one or both parents or a sibling), indicate exclusive
breastfeeding for at least 4 months has a protective effect.

Practice points: atopy

- In infants with a family history of atopy, maternal avoidance of
  specific foods such as milk, dairy products, eggs and peanuts
  during pregnancy and lactation has not been proven to be
  effective in reducing the incidence and severity of atopy in
  infants, compared with exclusive breastfeeding without
  maternal food restriction.
- Restricted diets, particularly during pregnancy, are not
  recommended.
- For the occasional, exclusively breastfed infant who may
  develop allergic responses due to the passive transfer of food
  antigens from the mother's diet through breast milk, a trial
  elimination diet of suspect foods (e.g. cows' milk, fish, eggs,
  soy and peanuts) can be considered, but this requires clinical or
  dietetic supervision.

Enhanced cognitive development. Cohort studies show children who
were breastfed have slightly higher cognitive development than bottle-
fed infants. There are many candidate factors in breast milk, such as

hormones and LCPUFAs, that theoretically might promote neuro-development. However, interpretation of published data is complicated because breastfeeding is associated with higher socioeconomic status and education, and more positive health behaviors. In some studies the benefits have been found even after attempts to take such demographic differences into account; in other studies they have not. The evidence in premature babies, in whom formal study is more feasible, and in whom brain development is perhaps at a more vulnerable stage, indicates that cognitive benefits from breast-milk feeding are plausible.

Effects on long-term cardiovascular risk. Observational studies have indicated that breastfed babies may be less prone to cardiovascular disease or its risk factors (such as high blood pressure) in later life. One randomized trial in preterm infants showed that those fed breast milk rather than formula in the neonatal period had lower diastolic and mean blood pressures 13–16 years later.

Other proposed benefits, which are less well defended scientifically, include reduced incidence of sudden infant death syndrome (SIDS), insulin-dependent diabetes mellitus (IDDM) and lymphoma. These associations could imply a possible 'programming' effect of breastfeeding on the development of the immune system, but further studies are needed.

Potential contraindications to breastfeeding

Breastfeeding is recommended for all infants, with very few exceptions. The recommendations concerning drugs in breast milk and the treatment of maternal infections are summarized in Tables 4.3 and 4.4. Important contraindications include HIV, untreated maternal tuberculosis and galactosemia in the infant, because galactose is a product of milk sugar (lactose) digestion. The estimated risk of transmission of HIV through breast milk by a woman during the viremic phase is 29%; the risk is 14% when the mother was already HIV antibody-positive during pregnancy.

There is no current justification to restrict breastfeeding due to environmental contaminants. Recent reports continue to document high accumulation of polychlorinated dibenzo-*p*-dioxins (PCDDs) and dibenzofurans (PCDFs) in breast milk. Although there is evidence of

TABLE 4.3

Drugs and the breastfed baby

- Most prescription drugs do not constitute a significant risk but, if uncertain, refer to the literature or information service on any drug given to a lactating mother
- Contraindications to breastfeeding include:
  - long-term chemotherapy
  - radioisotopes (stop breastfeeding for 1–2 weeks depending on the isotope used)
  - bromocriptine, cyclophosphamide, doxorubicin, ciclosporin, ergotamine, lithium, methotrexate, phencyclidine
  - illegal 'hard' drugs
- Use herbal remedies with caution, as some may contain active ingredients
- Alcohol may reduce milk intake, and sustained habitual drinking (i.e. > 2 units/day) in the first 3 months may affect motor development in the infant
  - occasional drink acceptable
  - if several drinks taken, postpone breastfeeding for 1 hour/unit of alcohol if possible

TABLE 4.4

Maternal infections and breastfeeding

Infection	Recommendation
HIV-antibody positive	Alternatives to breastfeeding indicated unless infant is also HIV-antibody positive at birth
Tuberculosis (active)	Breastfeeding indicated only after the mother has received adequate therapy and is considered to be non-infectious
Cytomegalovirus	Not a contraindication to breastfeeding
Rubella	Not a contraindication to breastfeeding
Acquired hepatitis B during nursing	Prompt immunization with hepatitis B vaccine and continue breastfeeding
Herpes simplex on or near nipple	Stop breastfeeding until lesion healed

short-term adverse neurodevelopmental outcomes with prenatal exposure to polychlorinated biphenyls (PCBs), no long-term developmental effects have been reported and, overall, breastfed infants have higher cognitive performance than those fed formula. Smoking and occasional alcohol usage are not contraindications to breastfeeding.

General recommendations to encourage breastfeeding

Breastfeeding is the optimal method of feeding infants. It may continue for up to 2 years or more and should be encouraged for at least the first 4–6 months.

In modern society, women now have limited opportunity to learn about breastfeeding in the traditional way by observing other breastfeeding mothers. If breastfeeding is to be promoted, health professionals need to play an active role to improve its uptake and duration (Table 4.5). Key elements in encouraging breastfeeding are:

TABLE 4.5

Ways to encourage and support breastfeeding

- Develop a local policy for advising and assisting breastfeeding mothers
- Provide antenatal and postnatal counseling on the benefits and practice of breastfeeding
- Ensure new mothers have actually seen breastfeeding (e.g. in antenatal classes)
- Ensure availability of experienced staff to give advice and assistance on normal breastfeeding and deal with breastfeeding problems
- Encourage frequent feeds (on demand) including night-feeds during the early postnatal period – do not suggest time limits or limit the number of feeds
  - start feeds soon after birth
  - more breastfeeding will increase the release of prolactin and therefore milk production
- Use no other 'top-up' fluids, such as water, glucose water or formula, unless indicated on clinical grounds (e.g. hypoglycemia)
- Ensure community support for mothers discharged home early

- education and counseling on health benefits
- use of active public health policies that have been shown to be effective
- avoidance of medical policies, for example time restriction of feeds, that interfere with successful lactation.

In European countries where breastfeeding rates are highest (Scandinavia) there has been political support for breastfeeding with prolonged maternity leave (e.g. 6 months) and paternity leave.

Use of breast milk in preterm infants

Recent data show human milk has particular importance for premature babies. These infants are too immature to be suckled, and mothers need to express their milk. Mothers should be actively counseled and assisted to provide breast milk for these infants even if they do not propose to breastfeed and can only manage to provide a proportion (preferably at least 30%) of their infant's milk needs for the first few weeks.

Human milk does not meet the nutritional needs of smaller preterm infants and requires supplementation. Nevertheless, inclusion of human milk in the diet (either the mother's own milk or milk donated to a milk bank) may reduce serious morbidity and mortality in preterm infants, improve long-term cognitive function and reduce blood pressure later in life. Current evidence for such benefits provides a basis for counseling (Table 4.6).

TABLE 4.6

Potential advantages of breastfeeding for the preterm infant

- Reduced incidence and improved prognosis of necrotizing enterocolitis
- Reduced incidence of systemic sepsis, even in Western neonatal units
- Improved feed tolerance with a more rapid escalation to full feeds and a reduced requirement for parenteral nutrition
- Higher cognitive and motor performance at follow-up
- Cardiovascular benefits – lower blood pressure, LDL cholesterol and insulin resistance at follow-up in adolescence

Nutritional recommendations for breastfed babies

Breastfed infants should receive breast milk exclusively for the first 4–6 months. WHO recently suggested that introduction of weaning food should be delayed until 6 months (rather than 4–6 months as previously recommended). In our view, insufficient scientific evidence supports such a recommendation for developed countries, though it is justified in developing countries where water supplies may be contaminated and weaning foods are often of poor quality. No other fluids, for example water, are required, even in moderately hot environments. In the USA, juice is not recommended before 6 months (see Chapter 6, page 53).

Maternal diet. Nutritional supplementation of mothers has a variable effect on breast milk. Macronutrient levels are affected little, except in maternal malnutrition. Levels of minerals (e.g. iron) and fat-soluble vitamins (A, D, E, K) in breast milk are minimally influenced by recent maternal diet, since they can be drawn from body stores. However, the types of fat consumed may affect breast-milk fatty acid profile and the levels of the water-soluble vitamins (C and B complex) in the maternal diet readily influence breast-milk content. Nevertheless, providing the mother is well nourished, supplementation is unnecessary. If she eats a very restricted diet (e.g. vegan), supplemental nutrients (e.g. vitamin B_{12}) help to ensure adequate nutrient delivery to her breastfed infant.

Nutritional supplementation of breastfed infants. Except for vitamins K and D, fluoride (see Chapter 7, page 57) and the introduction of iron-rich foods from around 5 months, vitamin and mineral supplementation of breastfed term infants in the first 6 months is not recommended. The addition of complementary foods from 4–6 months is discussed in Chapter 7.

Vitamin K levels are low in breast milk (around 2 µg/mL), but are higher in colostrum ($\leq$ 5 µg/mL). In contrast, non-supplemented formulas usually contain around 6–11 µg/mL and supplemented formulas up to 100 µg/mL. Parenteral prophylaxis against hemorrhagic disease with vitamin K, 1 mg, at birth is effective and routinely administered to newborn infants. Oral vitamin K has been considered, but a single oral dose provides insufficient vitamin K stores to protect breastfed infants reliably against hemorrhagic disease beyond the neonatal period. Therefore, multiple oral doses are needed, with the consequent problems of compliance. Late hemorrhagic disease of breastfed infants has been reported even after three oral doses, although 12 or more doses appear effective. Therefore it makes more sense to use a single parenteral dose of vitamin K.

Vitamin D. Three factors influence the vitamin D status of an infant:
- vitamin D status at birth
- vitamin D intake
- exposure to sunlight.

Poor maternal vitamin D status during pregnancy reduces the vitamin D status of an infant at birth. Women with little exposure to sunlight and who do not consume foods fortified with vitamin D or take vitamin supplements are at increased risk of vitamin D deficiency. In addition, infants at greatest risk of deficiency are those who are exclusively breastfed, are not exposed to sunlight or are dark-skinned; cholecalciferol (vitamin D) is synthesized in the skin from 7-dehydrocholesterol under the influence of sunlight. Breast milk is not a dependable source of vitamin D; poor maternal vitamin D status during lactation further reduces vitamin D in breast milk. Because it is not possible to identify all infants at risk of vitamin D deficiency, which has acute and long-term serious sequelae that are totally preventable, supplements of 5–10 µg or 200–400 IU daily are prudent for breastfed full-term infants. Such supplementation is low risk and should continue until the diet provides a source of vitamin D.

5 Infant formulas and other milks

What are infant formulas?

Earlier this century 'infant formulas' resembled cows' milk. Since the mid-1970s, following problems with older formulas (Table 5.1), highly adapted modern infant formulas were developed. Such formulas, based on the composition of mature human milk, no longer resemble cows' milk. The fats have been replaced with vegetable oils, proteins have been engineered to adjust the casein:whey ratio, mineral contents have been radically altered (e.g. phosphorus has been decreased because it depresses calcium levels, leading to convulsions, while iron has been greatly increased), and there has been substantial micronutrient fortification. The field has developed rapidly and numerous specialized formulas for specific uses have been developed. With advances in biotechnology and increased understanding of breast-milk biology, new additions to formulas have occurred or are being researched including taurine, carnitine, long-chain polyunsaturated fatty acids (LCPUFAs), nucleotides and oligosaccharides. Novel research, for instance in transgenic animals, may make it possible, if proven desirable, to add biologically active factors found in breast milk.

Formula quality control

Cows' milk is not recommended for babies in their first year. Consequently, infant formula is now the food most commonly used to feed Western infants, even those initially breastfed, since most mothers

TABLE 5.1

Adverse effects of cows' milk and older formulas

- Convulsions due to mineral imbalance
- Hypertonic dehydration during diarrheal states
- Iron-deficiency anemia
- Rickets and scurvy

cease to breastfeed exclusively well before 1 year. Given the dominance of infant formula in the diet together with our new appreciation of the importance of early nutrition, standards of formula design and testing have been regulated to the point that clinical efficacy and safety trials are now conducted with the stringency associated with pharmaceutical studies. Infant formula cannot mimic breast milk; the modern objective is to attempt to design products that induce in the infant a physiological response as close as possible to that of the breastfed baby.

Cows'-milk-protein-based formulas

Formulas based on cows' milk protein are the standard for healthy term infants who are not being breastfed. These formulas are fortified with iron and contain similar amounts of nutrients (protein, fat, minerals, trace minerals and vitamins) to those in mature human milk. Although not recommended for routine use, low-iron formulas are available in North America and some other countries, based on quite unsubstantiated concerns that iron in regular formula might cause constipation and other problems. In babies not breastfed, an iron-fortified formula should be used until an infant is 12 months old and consuming a variety of foods. At this time, formula can be replaced with pasteurized whole milk.

Soy-protein-based formulas

Up to 10% of infants in the UK and as many as 25% of infants in the USA use soy-protein-based formulas, presumably because of a perceived or real intolerance to cows' milk. All soy formulas sold are fortified with iron. Soy formulas have had a number of problems over the years, which have now been addressed (e.g. low contents of chloride, iodine and methionine, and high phytate content). The high content of aluminum in soy formulas compared with breast milk has been raised as a theoretical concern, though this aluminum has not been shown to be excessively absorbed or deleterious. The presence of plant estrogens (phytoestrogens) in soy formula has received much scientific and media attention. Reassuringly, recent follow-up in adulthood of over 800 subjects in infant feeding studies in Iowa, USA, between 1967 and 1978 showed no difference between those fed soy versus cows'-milk-based formula for over 30 later outcomes of current interest, including reproductive health.

Despite the widespread use of soy formulas, indications are limited. Apart from their use in infants on vegan diets and in rare cases of galactosemia, soy formulas are primarily employed in the dietary management of infants with proven allergy to cows' milk. Their use in the *prevention* of atopy is controversial. Evidence demonstrating a reduced prevalence of atopic diseases in high-risk infants (with a positive family history) fed soy-protein-based formulas in the first 6 months of life is not convincing. For some infants, there is cross-reactivity between cows'-milk-protein-based and soy-protein formulas. Approximately 30–40% of infants at risk of atopic disease will be sensitized to soy protein, particularly if the small bowel is damaged. For infants at high risk of, or with documented allergy to, cows'-milk protein, the formula of first choice is a whey or casein hydrolysate (see below).

Specialized infant formulas

Some specialized infant formulas (Table 5.2), including those for preterm infants and for dietary management of very specific medical conditions (such as phenylketonuria) are available only through hospital pharmacies. Other specialized infant formulas are available at the retail level and are intended for subgroups of infants with special nutrient needs or those who cannot tolerate entire cows'-milk-protein-based or soy-protein-based formulas (medical advice is recommended).

Lactose-free, cows'-milk-protein-based formulas are suitable for infants with lactose intolerance, although this is extremely rare until well after the weaning period, even in non-Caucasians. Because such formulas may contain residual galactose, they are contraindicated for infants with galactosemia. They contain the same ingredients as other infant formulas based on cows' milk, except that glucose polymers from corn syrup solids are substituted for lactose. They may be useful during periods of secondary disaccharidase deficiency due to acute enteritis or chronic conditions affecting the integrity of the small intestine, such as diarrhea and enteropathies.

TABLE 5.2

Commonly used specialized infant formulas

Intended use	Special features
Allergy avoidance (hydrolysed or partially hydrolysed proteins)	Do not contain whole proteins
Intestinal malabsorption	Contain simple sugars (glucose polymers), readily absorbed fats (medium-chain triglycerides) and hydrolysed or partially hydrolysed proteins
Lactose intolerance	Lactose-free
Anti-reflux formulas	Contain thickening agents claimed to reduce gastric reflux
Preterm formulas	Nutrient-enriched to achieve rapid rates of growth that would have occurred in utero; higher in protein, energy and minerals
Post-discharge preterm formulas	Specialized formulas for use after hospital discharge, which conform to guidelines for full-term formulas, but towards the higher end of accepted levels of nutrients, notably protein and minerals, needed to promote catch-up growth

Protein hydrolysate formulas are termed partially or extensively hydrolysed, depending on the extent of hydrolysis and ultrafiltration to which they have been subjected. Allergenicity lessens with more extensive hydrolysis and filtration.

- Extensively hydrolysed formulas (currently casein-, whey- or soy-based) are intended for feeding infants who have confirmed allergy to cows' milk or soy proteins. These formulas are quite costly.
- Partially hydrolysed formulas (currently whey-based) are intended for feeding infants at high risk for allergy. These formulas are more palatable and less expensive.

Despite cost and palatability, some experts would still choose the extensively hydrolysed formulas for prevention of allergy. Although in some trials, casein hydrolysate formulas have been found to be significantly less allergenic than whey hydrolysate formulas, which in turn are less allergenic than ordinary cows'-milk formulas, there have still been reports of reactions to whey and casein hydrolysates in highly allergic infants. While the most extensively hydrolysed protein formulas should be used for infants with allergy, some caution is still indicated. Such formulas may pose problems with palatability.

Follow-on formulas

Follow-on formulas are an alternative to standard infant formulas in the second 6 months of life when infants are already eating solid foods. Compared with cows' milk, follow-on formulas provide more appropriate quantities and forms of nutrients, including essential fatty acids, which are better absorbed during this transition period. They provide a lower renal solute load and have been shown to promote better iron status. However, no superiority of follow-on formulas to standard formulas has been established.

Current and future issues in infant formula design

In recent years, infant formula manufacturers have sought to improve their products by conducting research on the efficacy and safety of adding specific bioactive ingredients. This, together with increasing evidence that even small differences between formulas can have a significant effect on the infant, emphasizes that infant formulas cannot now be regarded as 'all the same'. There is now an onus on healthcare professionals to evaluate carefully information on individual products in order to give informed advice. Some examples of areas under research are given here.

Long-chain polyunsaturated fatty acids. Modern formulas contain the essential fatty acids, linoleic and α-linolenic acid, which can be metabolized to produce long-chain polyunsaturated fatty acids (LCPUFAs). Two such LCPUFAs, arachidonic acid (AA) and docosahexaenoic acid (DHA), are essential components of the brain and retina. The presence of AA and DHA in human milk but not in formulas containing vegetable oils has raised questions about whether the formula-fed infant would be able to synthesize adequate amounts endogenously to support normal development. There have been compelling biochemical data on higher DHA levels in blood and brain in breastfed versus formula-fed infants. The earlier clinical studies that attempted to determine the need for a dietary source or for the addition of AA and DHA to infant formulas were too small, yielded inconsistent results, assessed limited outcomes, did not incorporate sufficient follow-up or did not address safety adequately. However, accumulating evidence from more modern, larger studies shows that LCPUFA supplementation in full-term and particularly in preterm infants may be beneficial, at least in the short term, for cognitive and visual development. LCPUFAs are now being incorporated increasingly into infant formulas. There is still much ongoing research to evaluate the health consequences of LCPUFA intake in both preterm and full-term infants. As further research is published, the ultimate role of LCPUFAs in infant nutrition will become apparent.

Nucleotides. Some formulas contain added nucleotides in amounts based on the content in breast milk. Nuclcotides, which are the building blocks of nucleic acids (RNA and DNA) have numerous biological roles, notably their effects on the immune system. Their incorporation into formulas may reduce the incidence of diarrhea, enhance the immunological response to vaccination (e.g. with *Haemophilus influenzae* B) and promote growth.

Palmitic acid (C16:0) accounts for over 25% of breast-milk fat. Although formulas also contain palmitic acid (from vegetable oils), its position in the triglyceride molecule differs from that in breast milk (Figure 5.1), and this affects its handling in the gut. Experimental studies show that palmitate in the 1 and 3 positions has multiple effects on the infant, including reduced palmitate absorption, reduced fat absorption, reduced calcium absorption and bone mineral content, and an increase in formation of insoluble calcium soaps in the gut, leading to harder stools and, in premature infants, increased risk of intestinal obstruction due to inspissated calcium soaps. However, the long-term health consequences are unknown and currently under investigation.

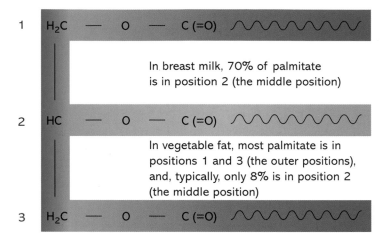

Figure 5.1 Palmitic acid in fats. The diagram represents a triglyceride with a glycerol backbone and three fatty acids in positions 1, 2 and 3.

Practical aspects of formula feeding

Detailed instructions for reconstitution of artificial feeds and the hygienic use of feeding utensils can be obtained from manufacturers, but the following points must be emphasized with regard to the safe and effective use of infant formulas:

- Infant formulas may be provided in the form of 'ready to feed' sterile liquid (commonly used by hospitals for convenience and in widespread use in the USA) or as powder (less expensive and more commonly used worldwide). When powdered milk is used, the quality of water added is important (see Chapter 6, page 53).
- Following concerns over the dangers of over- or underconcentration of infant feeds due to inaccurate reconstitution from powder, measuring scoops are now made at least as wide as their depth, reducing error, and manufacturers have cooperated to standardize scoops (one scoopful for each 30 mL or 1 fl oz of water). Nevertheless, there are still inherent difficulties in accurately dispensing milk powder, and recent data show significant deviations from recommended nutrient concentrations in milks made up by mothers. Therefore, parents must be appropriately advised on the careful preparation of milk from powder.

Water

Water used for preparing infant formulas and other foods, or for drinking, must be 'safe', that is free of microbiological and chemical contamination. Tap water, well water (that meets safety standards) and commercially bottled water (except carbonated or mineral water) are generally suitable for infant feeding (Table 6.1), but none is sterile. To ensure pathogen-free water for infants under 4 months, water should be brought to a rolling boil for at least 2 minutes. Boiled water can be stored refrigerated for 2–3 days in a sterilized, tightly closed container, or for 24 hours at room temperature in a sterile container.

Tap water. In most countries, municipal drinking water systems are routinely inspected and monitored for chemical and microbiological quality. Water from the cold water tap should be used, since hot water can dissolve or leach more lead and other non-biological contaminants. To flush any build-up of contaminants such as lead and copper, which tend to accumulate in water pipes overnight, the water should be

TABLE 6.1

Types of water*

Water type	Recommendations for infant feeding
Tap	Usually safe, but use from cold water tap
Well	Use with caution as it may contain a high content of nitrates, fluoride and other heavy metals
Bottled	
Non-carbonated	Safe if from springs and treated, and if low in mineral content
Carbonated	Unacceptable levels of carbon dioxide, sodium nitrate and fluoride; should not be used for infants

*None of these is sterile

allowed to run freely for about 2 minutes every morning. Many houses are still supplied by lead pipes and soft water is particularly plumbosolvent. The 1999 WHO guidelines recommend that the lead content of water used to make up formula feeds should not exceed 10 µg/liter (48.3 nmol/liter).

Well water. Caution is indicated, because well water may have naturally high concentrations of nitrates, nitrites, arsenic, fluoride or heavy metals. It should be tested for these, as well as coliform bacteria, at least twice a year. Water containing more than 10 parts per million (ppm) of nitrate is a health hazard for infants, since it may cause methemoglobinemia, particularly between 3–6 months of age. Nitrates are not eliminated by boiling water. Water containing more than 1.5 ppm of fluoride may cause dental fluorosis (mottled staining of the teeth) and should not be used.

Commercially bottled waters suitable for infants include non-carbonated natural spring water from underground springs and treated water (low mineral content).

Commercially bottled waters unsuitable for infants include mineral water, treated water with a high mineral content and carbonated water, including club soda. These waters may contain unacceptable levels of carbon dioxide, sodium, nitrate and fluoride.

There are no clear indications for the use of distilled water.

Home water-treatment equipment is not without risk. Some water softeners increase the sodium content of the water, and charcoal filters can leach silver or may contaminate the water with bacteria. The suitability of individual home water-treatment equipment may be determined by contacting the appropriate water authority.

Fruit juices

Juice is not an essential part of the infant's diet, yet its perceived value as a 'health food' results in excessive and widespread use. Up to a few ounces per day for older infants should be regarded more as a 'treat' than as a basic dietary ingredient. Breast milk, infant formula, and vegetables and whole fruits can easily provide the recommended intake of vitamin C, 50 mg daily.

Excessive juice consumption might indirectly contribute to inadequate intakes of more suitable foods, notably milk, and hence reduce nutrient and energy intake. Because of the sorbitol and fructose content of fruit juices, excessive intake may cause diarrhea, poor weight gain and failure to thrive. The risk of diarrhea is increased with certain juices. A recent study showed less carbohydrate malabsorption with sorbitol-free white grape juice than clear apple juice. Excessive fruit juice intake may also promote dental caries and nursing bottle syndrome.

Practice point: juice

- The UK Department of Health does not regard juice as necessary in an infant's diet, and the American Academy of Pediatrics does not recommend it for infants under 6 months of age.

Other beverages

Beverages containing caffeine and theobromine are inappropriate for infants (Table 6.2). Caffeine and theobromine are stimulants found in coffee, tea, some carbonated beverages such as colas, and hot chocolate. Importantly, tea reduces iron absorption. Sodas, fruit drinks,

TABLE 6.2

Beverages inappropriate for infant feeding

Beverage	Reason for poor suitability
Coffee, tea, colas	High in caffeine and theobromine
Sodas, fruit drinks, sport drinks	High in sugar, which may increase risk of dental caries
Herbal teas	May contain pharmacologically active, 'toxic' substances, and have no nutrient value

punches and sport drinks are also not recommended for infants because of their high sugar content and lack of nutrients other than carbohydrates. These drinks may also increase the risk of dental caries and nursing bottle syndrome.

Herbal teas. A recent trend towards the use of 'natural' substances and alternative medicine has increased interest in herbs and herbal teas. Toxic effects of herbal teas have been reported in an infant, and in two breastfed newborns whose mothers were drinking large amounts of herbal tea mixture. Usually there is no requirement to label herbal preparations used by adults with regard to their suitability for infants, yet there is insufficient information on safety.

Managing weaning, that is the introduction of solid foods to a hitherto exclusively milk-fed infant, is an important part of parenting. Specific weaning foods (transitional or complementary) are chosen to:

- satisfy hunger
- promote enjoyment of the taste of food and the social aspects of eating
- meet nutrient requirements for optimal growth, development and health
- prevent nutrient deficiencies (e.g. iron deficiency)
- minimize the risk of food allergies
- prevent major adult diseases including heart disease, diabetes, obesity, stroke and osteoporosis, which may be influenced by diet in early life.

The first two reasons could be labeled as social or pleasurable, and the last four as health-related. It is not yet clear if these diverse and potentially contradictory reasons for eating can be reconciled. Most research on infant nutrition has focused on the first 6 months; weaning has received relatively little scientific attention, particularly with regard to possible long-term health effects.

Timing of the transition

A successful transition from breast milk or formula to table food depends on appropriate timing in terms of the infant's nutritional needs and developmental readiness. It has been suggested that early introduction of weaning foods may increase the risk of infections and allergy, and perhaps even predispose to later obesity or cardiovascular disease, though this is speculative. Nevertheless, delayed weaning carries the risk of:

- faltering growth (wasting and stunting)
- specific nutrient deficiencies (e.g. energy, iron, zinc and vitamin D)
- development of feeding problems, including reliance on fluids and refusal to progress to textured foods.

The process of weaning should begin when breast milk or infant formula alone is insufficient to meet nutrient needs. Weaning practices vary in different cultures and geographic regions. Nevertheless, by 4–6 months of age, breast milk alone ceases to meet the infant's nutritional needs and weaning foods are required (see below). At this stage, sufficient physiological, developmental and behavioral maturation has occurred for introduction of solids (Tables 7.1 and 7.2).

Nutritional needs during the transition period

Transitional (weaning) foods are first introduced to meet nutrient and energy needs that are no longer totally met by breast milk (see Table 3.3, page 32).

Protein and energy. Breast-milk intake rises to a peak by 4 months, providing a mean of 750–850 mL/24 hours (range 500–1200 mL/24 hours and more in boys than girls). At this stage, typical intakes of 150 mL/kg body weight provide 1.5 g protein/kg/day and 85–105 kcal/kg/day. Beyond this age, protein and energy intakes per kilogram fall as the infant grows, and eventually, without

TABLE 7.1

Physiological factors facilitating the introduction of solid foods at 4–6 months

- The digestive system has developed sufficiently to permit good absorption of a variety of foods

- The 'extrusion reflex' useful for sucking and fixing the nipple in the mouth has gradually disappeared

- The secretion of saliva has increased and facilitates the swallowing of solid foods

- Neuromuscular coordination has improved; the tongue is now able to pass solids from the front to the back of the mouth

- The mucosal barrier has matured and the risk of food allergies has diminished

- Head control has improved; the infant can sit up, lean forward, turn away and send cues of satiety to the caregiver

transitional weaning foods, breast milk alone will be insufficient. The point at which this occurs is variable and difficult to define even for populations. The recommended dietary allowance (RDA) for protein, which is about 2 g/kg/24 hours in infancy, has an inbuilt safety margin, and it is now recognized that the RDA for energy (e.g. 116 kcal/kg/24 hours at 3 months) is unrealistically high compared with much lower intakes of breastfed babies growing and developing normally.

The traditional approach to assessing the adequacy of the diet is to monitor growth and watch for centile crossing. However, healthy breastfed babies, who are being fed in accordance with present-day practices, do not grow according to previously established growth standards, notably the US National Center for Health Statistics (NCHS) growth standard, which was based largely on formula-fed infants. Data from several countries show a marked secular trend in growth performance with the recent resurgence of breastfeeding. Typically in the first 3 months, the breastfed baby gains weight and length at a relatively fast rate so that the centiles are above the NCHS values. However, beyond 4 months there is a progressive deceleration of growth, a process which persists throughout infancy, despite weaning; indeed modern breastfed infants may remain leaner than those fed formula up to 18 months, and some data suggest they remain lighter and shorter up to pre-school age.

Whether these data indicate that breast milk is an inadequate sole source of nutrition beyond 4 months (on average) or rather that new standards are required to accommodate the growth pattern of breastfed babies is debated. The new British growth standards (see Chapter 3, page 23) go some way towards the latter, by including growth data from modern breastfed babies. In the absence of long-term outcome data on the consequences of these different early growth patterns, most authorities accept that exclusive breastfeeding provides adequate protein and energy for growth at least up to 4 months and that transitional foods will have to be introduced some time between 4 and 6 months. The recent WHO recommendation (see page 44) that breastfed infants should not generally receive any complementary foods before the age of 6 months has not been universally accepted by Western doctors, many of

TABLE 7.2

Development, feeding and communication skills, and food choices

Periods of infant feeding	Physical development	Feeding skills
Nursing *Newborn*	• Poor control of head, neck and trunk • Most movements are random and reflexive: randomly moves arms and legs; reflexively 'mouths' hands and toys	• Roots in search of nipple • Can suck and swallow only liquids • Holds liquids in mouth with help of fat pads in cheeks
Transitional *Head up*	• Doubles birth weight and weighs at least 6 kg/13 pounds • Emerging postural stability and trunk control; sits with help; when placed on stomach, lifts head and supports weight with straight arms • Newborn reflexes diminish • Purposely bats objects with fists; deliberately mouths hands and toys	• Opens mouth as spoon approaches • Quickly learns to suck thin purées from spoon • Uses tongue to move food to the back of the mouth to swallow without gagging
Sitter	• Good postural stability; sits alone • Developing independent mobility: rolls from back to front and 'creeps' on stomach • Emerging hand skills: rakes small objects towards self into a fist, transfers objects from one hand to the other	• Easily eats a variety of thin purées • Learns to keep thick purées in mouth and swallow without gagging • Begins drinking from a lidded cup with assistance
Crawler	• Strong postural stability: can reach out for a toy without losing balance • Improving mobility: crawls well; pulls self up to stand • Practicing hand skills: uses thumb and finger to hold small objects	• Uses tongue to move food to side of mouth for mashing • Holds lidded cup while drinking without help • Shows interest in feeding self by reaching out for utensils to mouth or play with them
Near-adult *Toddler*	• Tripled birth weight • Good mobility: walks with assistance; stands alone • Efficient hand skills: uses fingertips to delicately pick up small objects; reaches out with palms up to receive an object from someone else	• Keeps lips closed and most of food in mouth when chewing • Has some upper and lower teeth; bites through a variety of textured foods • Can easily feed self using fingers; learns to spear food with a fork and scoops with a spoon • Drinks from a cup; stops bottle feeding
Walker	• Masters gross motor skills • Walks with confidence • Masters fine motor skills: hand skills include a variety of grasp patterns; can manipulate objects within a hand; shows clear preference for one hand	• Uses lips, tongue and teeth to draw food and liquid into mouth for efficient eating • Uses one hand to adjust spoon into better position when scooping up a variety of consistencies • Can bring spoon to mouth with minimal spilling

Adapted from: Learning about Dietary Variety. *Pediatric Basics* 1994;69:4–5.

Communication skills	Food choices
• Cries and sucks intensely when hungry • Releases nipple or falls asleep during feeding when satisfied • Can regulate food intake to meet caloric needs by six weeks	• Breast milk
• Changes established feeding patterns. Seems hungry after actively breastfeeding 8–10 times a day, or drinking 950 mL/32 oz of formula • Moves forward as spoon approaches to signal hunger, pushes feeder's hand away when satisfied	• Breast milk or infant formula • Single-ingredient cereals and fine purées • Avoid foods containing egg, soy and wheat
• Grasps spoon as if to say 'I want that!' • Looks for food when feeding dish is removed	• Breast milk or infant formula • Thick purées • Mixed-ingredient foods, including egg, soy and wheat • Mild flavors
• Vocalizes, points or touches feeder's hand during mealtimes to control what and how much is being fed	• Breast milk or infant formula • Textures that encourage chewing • More complex seasonings and flavors
• Will mimic carers' mealtime behaviors • Uses words or sounds to express the desire for specific foods	• Introduce whole cows' milk when a sufficient variety of solid foods is being consumed • Foods with stronger flavors and varied textures for continued chewing practice
• Expresses mealtime wants with simple phrases, 'want that', 'more juice', 'all done' • Can lead carer to cupboard or refrigerator and point to a desired food or drink • Develops definite food preferences; may develop erratic eating behaviors	• Whole cows' milk • A wide variety of foods with challenging textures and flavors, as well as familiar favorites

whom favor a more individual approach. Until more outcome data are available, debate in this politically charged area will doubtless continue. However, regardless of the deliberations of committees and health professionals, babies themselves may play an important part in influencing the time of weaning by signaling their needs.

Iron. The requirement of breastfed infants for supplemental iron is controversial. Iron in breast milk is very well absorbed (around 80% compared with under 10% from fortified formulas) but levels are much lower than in modern formulas. A small proportion of breastfed infants have lower iron stores at 6 months, and a greater proportion appear deficient at 9 months or later, than those fed iron-supplemented formula.

Iron deficiency may impair neurodevelopment (though the evidence is incomplete) and immunity. Its prevalence varies depending on the socioeconomic and cultural group studied. In some ethnic groups (e.g. Asians in the UK) and in those from a deprived background, the incidence of iron-deficiency anemia in toddlers reaches 25–30%. This is a major community health concern. In bottle-fed infants, continued use of formulas fortified with iron and vitamin C during infancy is effective in preventing iron deficiency anemia, but in babies receiving breast milk plus weaning foods beyond 6 months, good nutritional advice is required. Iron from iron-fortified cereals may not be well absorbed. Heme iron, preferably from red meat, is ideal though often not consumed in sufficient quantities. Vitamin C will enhance iron absorption from a meal. Tea, given to some infants, depresses iron absorption. If there is any doubt about the sufficiency of iron intake it may be prudent to give supplemental iron, though careful instruction is required on the danger to the child and siblings of accidental iron overdosage. Since iron stores are proportional to body mass at birth, babies small for their gestational age may become iron-depleted well before 6 months (Table 7.3).

Multivitamins. In the UK, though not in the USA or Canada, it has been recommended that breastfed infants over 6 months of age and formula-fed infants receiving less than 500 mL of formula should

TABLE 7.3

Risk factors for developing iron-deficiency anemia

Young infants

- Premature birth
- Fetal growth retardation
- Low hemoglobin concentration at birth
- Frequent infections

Older infants

- Early and prolonged intake of cows' milk
- Low intake of meat
- Low intake of foods containing vitamin C
- Exclusively breastfed for longer than 6 months without an iron supplement

receive a daily supplement of vitamin A (200 µg), vitamin C (200 mg) and vitamin D (7 µg) as a combined preparation for 5 years. This is, however, the subject of debate. Others would reserve this policy for infants in whom there is doubt about dietary adequacy.

Fluoride is not a nutrient, although epidemiological studies demonstrate its role in preventing dental caries. It has both systemic and topical actions. Systemically, it acts on the teeth prior to eruption and is incorporated into the structure of the enamel, making it resistant to decay and limiting enamel demineralization. It also acts topically by promoting remineralization, and possibly through antibacterial effects. The relative roles of systemic versus topical fluoride are still debated. In areas where water supply is fluoridated (fluoride ion > 0.3 ppm), infants consuming reconstituted formulas will have an adequate intake, but the intake of breastfed babies will inevitably be low. The American Academy of Pediatrics has recommended a fluoride intake of 0.25 mg daily from 6 months to 3 years, but emphasizes the dangers (fluorosis) of exceeding this dosage when all sources are combined.

What solid foods?

First foods. During the transition to solid foods, and indeed throughout the first year, infants should continue to consume breast milk or iron-fortified formula as the sole milk source. Iron-containing foods are recommended as first foods. The sequence of introduction most often followed is iron-fortified infant cereal, then vegetables, fruits, and finally meat and alternatives, though this sequence is not evidence-based (see below) and varies between cultures (Table 7.4).

Because of a perception that the infant's relatively permeable intestinal tract would encourage uptake of foreign proteins provoking allergic reactions, it is customary to limit the allergenic load by using a single-grain cereal as the first food. The use of single foods makes it

TABLE 7.4

Weaning practices in different cultures*

Where	Food	Texture	How
Highland Peru	Porridge and family soup	Thin semisolid mixtures	Spoon- and finger-fed by mother or other caregiver
Poland	Juice, soup with rice gruel; later, gruel with puréed apple or cows' milk; then puréed meat and egg yolk	Thin semisolid mixtures	Spoon- and bottle-fed by parents and sometimes grandmothers
Philippines	Rice gruel (water from cooking rice and calamansi – lemon – juice); later, commercial cereal, banana, broth, potatoes, eggs, meat and vegetables	Thin semisolid mixtures	Bottle- and spoon-fed by mother
USA	Rice cereal mixed with breast milk and later with juice or other liquids	Liquid to thin semi-solid mixtures	Spoon-fed by parents or other caregiver
Yorubaland, Nigeria	Diluted fermented porridge, maize or sorghum	Thin semisolid mixtures	Spoon- and hand-fed by mother or grandmother

* Adapted from Bentley M, Rudzka-Kańtoch Z, Florentino RF et al. Feeding windows on the world. In *World Feeding Views* 1998;3:11.

easier to identify the cause of any allergic reaction, though the validity of this approach to those without an atopic family history is debated. The most commonly used first food is iron-fortified rice cereal. Gluten-containing foods are often introduced after 6 months because they are more likely to cause allergic reactions.

There is little benefit to adding infant cereals or other puréed foods to bottles containing formula or milk. In fact, an important reason for introducing solids is the developmental readiness of the infant for spoon-feeding and more textured foods. Sucking food or thick liquids through a nipple carries a risk of choking and aspiration. There is no convincing evidence that adding cereal to the bedtime bottle helps infants sleep through the night.

While the order of introduction of weaning foods is not evidence-based, it is common practice to introduce vegetables before fruits, because it is perceived that vegetables are better accepted when introduced first. Traditionally (and undesirably – see below), meat (and its alternatives) is the last of the food groups introduced. The foods in this group include meats, fish, poultry, cooked egg yolks, and alternatives such as well-cooked legumes and tofu. Milk products such as cottage cheese, other cheeses and yoghurt are also introduced at this time. Egg white, which contains at least 23 different glycoproteins, is not traditionally given in the USA to infants until 1 year of age to minimize any possible allergic reactions, though hard-boiled whole egg is considered suitable from 6 months in the UK.

The traditional late introduction of meats is not logical. Indeed, meats are an excellent and reliable source of iron (and protein) and in the authors' view should be introduced, in puréed form, earlier in the sequence.

Table foods. The transition to other solid foods, such as more textured purées, finger foods and table foods eaten by the rest of the family, takes place in the latter part of the second 6 months as infants become able to chew. Safe finger foods include bread crusts, dry toast, pieces of soft cooked vegetables and fruits, soft ripe fruit such as banana, cooked meat and poultry, and cheese cubes. At this time, most infants are developmentally ready to feed themselves and should be encouraged to

> **Practice points: introducing new foods**
>
> - Start with a small amount of each new food, about 1 teaspoon, and increase the amount as the infant becomes used to the food.
> - When introducing new foods, offer the food on a couple of different days as the infant gets accustomed to the new taste.
> - New foods should be introduced when the caregiver is feeling relaxed and unhurried, and when the baby is calm and happy. A tense atmosphere may make the infant reject both the food and the eating experience.
> - Advise the caregiver to try to recognize cues from their infant. If babies are hungry, they will appear excited by waving their hands and kicking their feet when food is presented. They will lean forward and open their mouths. If babies are not hungry, they will close their mouths and turn their heads away or fall asleep.
> - Do not force feed. As long as the baby is healthy and achieving normal growth, rejection of food is a normal response at times; the food may be tried again a few days or a week later. If the baby still does not want it or like it, let it be. If the baby is forced to eat foods that he or she does not like, poor eating habits and negative associations with food and mealtimes may develop. No food is irreplaceable. Find other nutritious foods that the child will enjoy.
> - Watch out for undesirable food reactions (e.g. rashes, diarrhea, general discomfort or irritability).

do so. By 1 year of age, ingestion of a variety of food daily from the four food groups is recommended (dairy products; breads and cereals; fruits and vegetables; meat, poultry and fish).

Home-prepared foods. Caregivers may prepare solid foods by puréeing cooked fresh or frozen foods. Previously, it was recommended that home-prepared carrots, spinach, turnip and beets, which could contain nitrates, should be avoided before 6 months because of the danger of methemoglobinemia. Very young infants may be particularly susceptible because fetal hemoglobin is more readily oxidized to methemoglobin than is hemoglobin. However, current feeding practices, with the later introduction of solid foods, are unlikely to cause methemoglobinemia even in susceptible infants (gastric pH > 4 and nitrate-reducing bacteria in the upper gastrointestinal tract).

Commercial baby foods. Modern commercial baby foods provide a safe and effective way of meeting full nutrient needs during the transition to table foods. They are sterile, provide low levels of nitrates, sugar and salt compared with adult foods, and also contain no additives. They are most useful during the early transitional stage before the infant graduates to family table foods.

Food has major health and safety implications for the general population and poses some special health issues in infancy.

Infection

Gastroenteritis. Morbidity associated with diarrheal illness in the industrialized world is very high. In the USA alone, roughly $1.5 billion is spent each year to provide evaluation and care for approximately 16 million episodes of diarrheal illness (mainly viral in origin) in children younger than 5 years. Worldwide, 4 million children die each year from gastroenteritis and resulting malnutrition.

Oral rehydration therapy (ORT), combining the use of oral electrolyte solutions (OES) with early refeeding, has proven safe and effective for restoring and maintaining hydration and electrolyte balance in infants with mild and moderate dehydration, including those with vomiting. It is important for clinicians to recognize clinically degrees of dehydration (Table 8.1).

OES containing calculated concentrations of carbohydrate, sodium, potassium and chloride promote fluid and electrolyte absorption, while juices, carbonated soft drinks, tea, sport drinks and broth do not. Human milk is well tolerated during diarrhea and may reduce its severity and duration; therefore, breastfeeding should continue throughout the diarrhea with additional fluids given as OES. Early and rapid refeeding should start as soon as rehydration is achieved and vomiting stops (ideally within 6–12 hours of beginning treatment) (Table 8.2). Infants treated with OES and early refeeding have reduced stool output, shorter duration of diarrhea and improved weight gain. Routine change to lactose-free or diluted feeds is unnecessary in well-nourished infants with mild-to-moderate gastroenteritis. The Canadian Paediatric Society Nutrition Committee has recently published recommendations on assessment, treatment and early refeeding in the management of childhood gastroenteritis (Figure 8.1).

TABLE 8.1

Clinical assessment of dehydration

Mild (< 5% loss of body weight)
- Decreased urine output
- Increased thirst
- Slightly dry mucous membranes

Moderate (5–10% loss of body weight)
- Abnormal skin turgor
- Sunken eyes
- Very dry mucous membranes
- Depressed anterior fontanelle

Severe (> 10% loss of body weight)
- Signs of moderate dehydration plus any of the following:
  - rapid, weak pulse/hypotension
  - cold extremities
  - oliguria/anuria, coma

TABLE 8.2

Simplified oral rehydration therapy protocol in mild-to-moderate dehydration

Assessment	Oral rehydration protocol	
	Mild dehydration (0–5%)	Moderate dehydration (5–10%)
1st hour	20 mL/kg/hour	20 mL/kg/hour
Next 6–8 hours	10 mL/kg/hour administered evenly	15–20 mL/kg/hour
8–24 hours*	Oral electrolyte solution as required; early refeeding	
> 24 hours*	Delayed refeeding only if severe vomiting	

*Infant reassessed at 4-hourly intervals

Practice points: gastroenteritis

- Dehydration accompanying infantile gastroenteritis should be treated with early oral rehydration and early refeeding strategies.

- Infants with gastroenteritis should be offered maintenance solution to prevent dehydration. Parents and daycare centers should keep maintenance solution to hand in anticipation of episodes of infectious diarrhea.

- OES and maintenance solutions and instructions in their use should be made available at reasonable costs.

- Medical facilities should have ORT protocols available for staff and patients.

- Antidiarrheal drugs, antibiotics and antiemetic therapy are rarely indicated in gastroenteritis in childhood and should be discouraged.

- Home-made oral rehydration solutions are discouraged since serious errors in formulation have occurred.

- Infants with mild-to-moderate dehydration should be treated under medical supervision with ORT in preference to intravenous rehydration.

- Infants with severe dehydration should initially be treated with intravenous or intraosseous rehydration.

- Breastfed infants with dehydration should be given ORT in conjunction with continued breastfeeding.

- Early refeeding should commence as soon as vomiting has resolved, approximately 6–12 hours.

- Non-lactose-containing formulas or milks may be used if diarrhea and abdominal cramps persist beyond the expected 5- to 7-day course, suggesting clinical lactose intolerance.

- Further initiatives to encourage ORT use by patients and professionals should be developed.

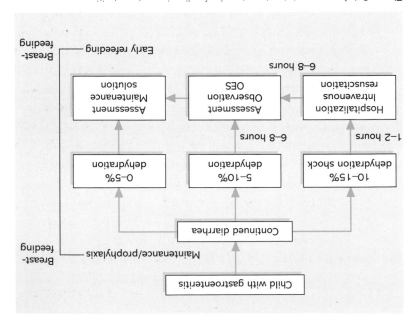

Figure 8.1 Assessment, treatment and refeeding in gastroenteritis.

Salmonellosis. *Salmonella* infection in childhood occurs in two major forms:

- gastroenteritis (including food poisoning), which may be very mild or severe and complicated by sepsis with or without focal suppurative complications
- enteric fever (typhoid and paratyphoid fever).

While the number of cases of typhoid fever has decreased, the incidence of *Salmonella* gastroenteritis has greatly increased in the past 15 years. Clinical features include fever, vomiting, diarrhea and polymorphonuclear leukocytosis with confirmation on stool (or blood) cultures. The highest incidence is seen in children under 6 years of age, with a peak at age 6 months to 2 years. Nursery epidemics have occurred, and infants under 6 months are very susceptible to complications.

The organisms are widespread in nature, infecting domestic and wild animals. Most non-human isolation of *Salmonella* is from poultry. The bacteria can occasionally be transmitted from infected hens directly into the eggs before the shells are formed.

Cracks in eggshells can allow transfer of bacteria to the egg contents. Contaminated egg powder and frozen whole-egg preparations used to make ice cream, custards and mayonnaise are often responsible for outbreaks. Transmission occurs primarily by ingestion of contaminated food. Since cooking destroys these bacteria, raw eggs and foods containing raw eggs should be avoided. Hygiene (handwashing and disinfecting food preparation surfaces) is needed when handling eggs.

Infant botulism. Honey is a risk factor for infant botulism and is the only food directly implicated. Surveys of random batches of honey indicated the normal range of *Clostridium botulinum* was approximately < 1–10 spores/kg, while honey implicated in infant botulism contained 10^3–10^4 spores/kg. There is a general consensus that honey should not be fed to children under 12 months. While earlier studies indicated the presence of low levels of *C. botulinum* in corn syrup, more recent studies have failed to confirm this, and corn syrups are now regarded as safe for babies.

Choking and aspiration

The risk of choking can be reduced if caregivers are aware of their toddler's chewing and swallowing abilities, supervise infants while eating, avoid offering foods with the potential to cause choking (Table 8.3), and know how to handle choking if it occurs.

The use of a 'propped bottle' to feed an unattended infant is not recommended because of the danger of choking or aspirating as the flow of milk into the mouth may be too rapid. The infant should sit upright while eating, and not lie down, walk, run or be distracted from the task of safe eating. Eating in a car is considered unsafe because if choking does occur, it is difficult to pull over to the side of the road safely. There is also an increased risk of choking if the car stops suddenly.

If choking does occur, there are a number of steps to follow, listed in Table 8.4. However, it is important to note the effectiveness of natural coughing. If a choking child can breathe and is able to speak and/or cough, all maneuvers are unnecessary and potentially dangerous.

TABLE 8.3

Reducing the risk of choking in infants and children under 4 years of age

Unsafe foods

- Popcorn
- Hard candies/sweets, gum, cough drops
- Raisins, peanuts or other nuts, and sunflower seeds
- Fish with bones
- Snacks using toothpicks or skewers

Safer foods

- Grated raw carrots or hard fruit pieces
- Fruits with pits removed and chopped
- Peanut butter spread thinly on crackers or bread*

*Peanut butter served alone, or on a spoon, is potentially unsafe because it can stick to the palate or posterior pharynx leading to asphyxia. Peanut preparations should not be given to infants less than 6 months of age

Food allergies

Adverse food reactions are generally divided into two categories:

- food intolerance
- food hypersensitivity.

An allergic reaction to a food involves the immune system. The incidence of food allergies has been estimated to be 2–10% in the first year of life, and decreases as children get older. The risk of developing food allergies is largely related to genetic predisposition and the age at which the food is introduced, with a greater risk of sensitization in the first year. Young infants are particularly prone because their immature intestinal system is more permeable to the absorption of food allergens and lacks local immune defenses. Most allergens are proteins of large molecular size. Food allergy commonly presents in infancy with the first introduction of whole cows' milk, egg or peanut, which, together with soy, nuts and wheat, are responsible for approximately 95% of food allergies in infants.

TABLE 8.4

Management of choking in infants (under 1 year of age)

Steps 1–5 should be repeated as needed and aid from the emergency medical services obtained as rapidly as possible

Step 1

Place the infant face down on the rescuer's forearm in a 60° head-down position with the head and neck stabilized. Rest the forearm firmly against the rescuer's body for additional support. If the infant is large, an alternative method is to lay the infant face down over the rescuer's lap, with the head firmly supported and held lower than the trunk

Step 2

Administer four back blows rapidly with the heel of the hand, high between the shoulder blades

Step 3

If the obstruction is not relieved, turn the infant over to a supine position and, resting on a firm surface, deliver four rapid chest thrusts (similar to external cardiac compressions) over the sternum using two fingers

Step 4

If breathing is not resumed, open the victim's mouth by grasping both the tongue and the lower jaw between the thumb and forefinger, and lift (the tongue-jaw lift technique); this draws the tongue away from the back of the throat and may help relieve the obstruction. If the foreign body can be seen, it may be manually extracted by a finger sweep. However, blind sweeps may cause further obstruction and thus should be avoided

Step 5

If no spontaneous breathing occurs, attempt ventilation with two breaths using a mouth-to-mouth or mouth-to-mouth and nose technique

It is rare for an infant to have allergies to more than two or three foods. In an exclusively breastfed infant, the source of allergens can be the mother's diet; proteins pass into the breast milk and are then ingested by the baby.

Diagnosis of food hypersensitivity requires a careful history to exclude other causes of adverse food reactions; selective skin-prick tests or radioallergosorbent tests (RAST) if an IgE-mediated disorder is suspected; appropriate removal of the food from the diet; and a subsequent challenge test under supervision.

Treatment of food hypersensitivity involves avoidance of foods proven to cause symptoms. Many food-related allergies disappear with age, usually before 4 years; re-challenging later with the offending food (with professional advice) is therefore recommended. Allergies to peanut, nuts, wheat, fish and seafood are the most severe and more likely to be lifelong. With multiple food allergies or severe food reactions, the assistance of an expert dietitian is advisable.

Practice points: food allergies

- Exclusion diets can result in significant nutritional deficiencies. Parents will need dietetic advice.
- Children with a family history of any atopy should not be fed foods containing peanuts before 3 years of age (UK recommendations).

Current interventions to actually prevent food hypersensitivity are not fully effective. Exclusive breastfeeding for at least 4 months has been shown to be helpful in infants at increased risk of food allergies. Studies using protein hydrolysate formulas and the delayed introduction of solid foods to prevent food hypersensitivity have been conflicting. A single recent study showed exclusive breastfeeding, or feeding a formula containing partially hydrolysed whey, was associated with a lower incidence of atopic disease and food allergy compared with feeding soy or conventional cows' milk formulas. Goats' milk is likely to be ineffective in preventing or treating cows' milk allergy since goats' and cows' milk proteins are so similar that 90% of babies allergic to cows' milk will be allergic to goats' milk.

Colic

Definition. Most babies presenting with 'colic' have what is perceived by parents as excessive crying. Infant crying behavior includes fussing (in most cases), crying, and less consolable intense crying. Using Wessels' rule of 3 – crying for more than 3 hours/day on at least 3 days/week for at least 3 weeks before the age of 3 months – around 25% of babies fulfill this criterion. Such crying generally occurs throughout the day, but is most prominent in the evening. Some have sought to distinguish this 'excessive crying' from 'colic', which should also include three of the following:

- paroxysmal episodes
- higher pitched, more intense cry during an episode
- hypertonia
- inconsolability.

If this distinction is accepted, 'colic' is a much less common phenomenon than excessive crying and applies to only a small proportion of babies.

Key issues. A number of questions about colic/excessive crying are now being addressed.

- Is it one phenomenon or more?
- Is it a normal developmental process, given that the average 6-week-old baby cries for 2 hours each day?
- Is it related in origin to the gut or feeding?
- Should it be regarded as an illness or a social phenomenon – and is it in fact treatable?

Current evidence. The cause(s) of colic are debated. Some evidence links colic/crying with the gut or feeding, for example: for some 'colicky' babies, switching from cows'-milk formula is effective; infants fed using an anti-vacuum feeding bottle to reduce air-swallowing have been shown to cry less; babies who grow faster cry more; and breastfed babies have been shown to cry less than formula-fed infants in the first month, but more in the second month.

Management. There are three general approaches:

- 'treat' the infant
- change the parent's interpretation of the infant's behavior
- change parental behavior.

Treatment of the infant has included strategies such as pharmacological agents, switching from cows'-milk-based formula, and the use of special feeding bottles, with variable success. The most researched drug is simethicone, a defoaming agent, but the most recent randomized, placebo-controlled, multicenter trial showed that it had no effect. Studies of herbal teas with possible antispasmodic activity have shown some initial promise, but safety has not been established.

Since infant crying or colic is self-limited (peaking at 6 weeks and resolved by 3–4 months) and excessive crying so common as to be almost regarded as 'normal', one approach is to educate mothers to 'expect' this to occur and not be overconcerned about any 'pathological' significance, though some infants will be intolerant of cows'-milk-based formula (which can be excluded) and occasionally infants with chronic crying will have organic pathology.

Parenting techniques may reduce infant crying or colic. Soothing, rocking, stroking, massaging, cuddling and motion (e.g. in a car) may be effective. In non-Western cultures frequent feeding and rapid response to the baby's distress appears to reduce the duration of crying (but not its occurrence or pattern). This suggests that excessive crying could, to some extent, be a product of Western parenting patterns.

Constipation and fiber

In infancy, clinically significant constipation is uncommon. There is wide variation in the 'normal' number of bowel movements each day, ranging from one after each feed to days apart. Bowel function is normal even when accompanied by straining and reddening of the face. There is no evidence that inadequate fluid or carbohydrate intake causes constipation in infants, nor that treating constipation with fruit juices or corn syrup is effective. Educating parents about the wide variation in normal bowel function seems essential to avoid the overtreatment or inappropriate treatment of normal variants.

Hard and painful bowel movements signal a mild-to-moderate problem in bowel function, whereas abdominal distension requires further work-up and medical intervention.

Increasing the fiber content of the diet may be helpful for infants over the age of 6 months, but a varied intake of fiber-containing foods (e.g. whole-grain breads and cereals, fruit and vegetables, cooked legumes) is suggested rather than the routine use of fiber supplements. There are no data to indicate the amount of fiber needed for normal laxation during the first 2 years of life. Recent recommendations on dietary fiber intake for children (age-plus-5 g daily) apply to children over the age of 2 years. These recommendations, to a large extent, reflect current dietary intake of fiber by children in North America. They are not based on evidence of disease prevention. There have been some nutrition-related concerns related to the excessive use of fiber, for example decreased growth and reduced nutrient bioavailability, though these concerns are poorly supported.

Dietary fat restriction

Fat is an important dietary component for the infant and toddler (Table 8.5). Energy and nutrient requirements are particularly high in the first 2 years of life. However, some parents believe that restriction of dietary fat in infancy is beneficial in reducing later cardiovascular disease. Dietary fat restriction can compromise energy, vitamin and essential fatty acid intake, and is not advised. There is no evidence that restricting fat intake during the first 2 years of life reduces illness in later life or provides benefit in childhood.

Nursing bottle syndrome

The etiology of nursing caries (Figure 8.2) is multifactorial and has been attributed in part to giving a bottle of sugar-containing beverage during sleep time or to pacify an infant, bottle-feeding after 12 months of age, the use of sweetened pacifiers and prolonged breastfeeding. Bathing teeth in nutrient-containing liquids (milk, fruit juices and fruit drinks, or carbonated, sugar-containing beverages) provides a continuous supply of nutritional substrate for dental bacteria to proliferate. This may result in carious teeth. When an infant is asleep, liquid can pool in the mouth, and salivary flow and oral cleaning are diminished. Children who fall asleep with a bottle in their mouth are at significantly greater risk of caries than infants who discard the bottle before falling asleep. The use of bottles or pacifiers dipped in sugar, syrup or honey during the day or night can also damage the infant's

TABLE 8.5

Importance of dietary fats

- Lipids are the predominant source of dietary energy for infants and young children, providing approximately 50% of the energy in human milk and a similar proportion in many formulas

- Dietary lipids slow gastric emptying and intestinal motility, and thereby may modulate the satiety value of food

- Dietary lipids provide essential polyunsaturated fatty acids and lipid-soluble vitamins

- Lipids are structural components in all tissues, particularly indispensable parts of all cell and plasma membrane systems

- The composition of structural lipids affects cell membrane functions, such as membrane fluidity, activity of membrane-bound enzymes and receptors, metabolite exchange and signal transduction. The brain and other neural tissues are particularly rich in structural lipids, and lipid supply and metabolism have been shown to affect neural function

- Some long-chain polyunsaturated fatty acids are precursors for bioactive lipid mediators, including prostaglandins, thromboxanes and leukotrienes. These eicosanoids are powerful regulators of numerous cell and tissue functions (e.g. thrombocyte aggregation, inflammatory reactions and leukocyte functions, vasoconstriction)

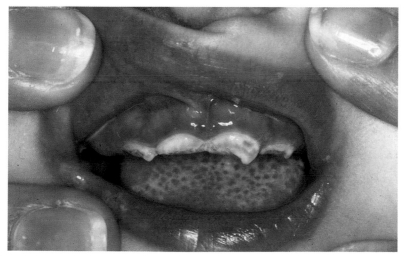

Figure 8.2 Tooth decay in an infant with feeding-bottle caries.

deciduous (primary) teeth. The effectiveness of preventative dental counseling in inducing dietary change has been questioned; however, for the prevention of nursing caries, it seems clinically sensible to counsel parents to avoid nocturnal and long-term use of baby bottles containing liquids other than water.

Vegetarian diets

With careful planning and advice, vegetarian diets for infants and children can be nutritionally adequate. For older infants, a carefully selected vegetarian diet can meet all the requirements of a growing child. Nutrient deficiencies that have been reported in vegetarian children include:

- iron
- vitamin B$_{12}$
- vitamin D
- energy.

Vegan diets

For vegan infants (those with no eggs, meat or dairy products in their diet), a commercially prepared soy infant formula is recommended during the first 2 years to improve provision of nutrients and energy for growth and development. Nevertheless, vegan babies are at significant risk for nutritional insufficiency, and parents will generally require supervision and skilled dietetic advice.

Feeding problems are common and diverse in origin. A logical approach to classification, initial decision-making, diagnosis and management is needed. Strictly, the term 'feeding problems' should apply to difficulties with the mechanics of feeding, but it is generally used more broadly to cover:

- underlying illness in the infant, presenting as a feeding problem
- problems with the mechanics of feeding
- problems apparently relating to the gut
- problems due to inappropriate feeding practices
- problems with feeding behavior and appetite
- maternal problems affecting infant feeding.

In this chapter we first present general considerations to guide assessment and management of feeding problems, mainly in the form of six key questions which professionals can ask themselves. Thereafter, we describe some specific problems as classified above.

General considerations to guide assessment and management

Assessment procedures involve some or all of the following steps.

- Take an obstetric and medical history. Past history is often relevant; for example, birth asphyxia can cause subtle neurological problems which can impair feeding, and prematurity can cause a broad range of feeding difficulties.
- Take a feeding history (Table 9.1).
- Take a full history of the feeding problem.
- Watch the child feeding (breast, formula or solids).
- Observe feed preparation by the mother (if relevant).
- Weigh and measure the child (see Chapter 3, page 23).
- Perform a medical examination.

Key questions. A systematic approach to assessment and management requires the professional to address the following questions.

TABLE 9.1

Taking an infant feeding history

- Types of feed used since birth
- Number of breast feeds and duration
- If formula-fed:
  - careful history of milk preparation and reconstitution
  - volume fed
- Volume of all fluids other than milk:
  - water
  - juice
  - other
- Quantities and types of weaning foods used
- Nutritional supplements
- Types of feeding vessels and utensils used
- Feeding behavior
- History of any feeding problems

Could this feeding problem be a manifestation of significant underlying illness? Bear in mind that significant and sometimes life-threatening illness requiring immediate attention can present as a feeding problem. Babies cannot verbalize their complaints. Major illness of a general systemic nature (e.g. infection, metabolic disturbance) or disease in specific organs (e.g. gut, heart, kidney, liver) can present in subtle ways, such as vomiting or lack of interest in food (see Table 9.2, page 86). Important clues to an underlying disease process include:
- an ill-looking baby
- drowsiness or apathy
- additional abnormal clinical signs.

If a baby with a feeding problem is unwell for no obvious reason, a medical examination is essential. The infant should be examined naked, and the assessment should include:
- overall appearance (skin tone, wasting, color, rashes)
- thorough examination of systems.

A cautionary case history is outlined below. While this is a relatively uncommon and unfortunate case, it serves to emphasize that:

- health professionals must appreciate the medical significance of some feeding problems
- vomiting should be appraised carefully – there are many important causes (see Table 9.2), and it should not necessarily be assumed that it points to a primary problem with the gut or feeding
- vomiting in an *unwell* child always deserves attention – in this case poor feeding with vomiting and drowsiness should have signaled that this was not a simple feeding problem.

> **It is critical that those advising on infant feeding and feeding problems are trained to recognize when a baby is ill** (see page 82).

Is there evidence of impaired nutrition? Feeding problems are more significant if associated with impaired nutritional status, which can be assessed by checking whether growth is faltering (see Chapter 3, page 23) and by taking a feeding history (Table 9.1). If so, this generally requires medical assessment and sometimes special investigations (see page 34).

Is this really a medical problem? Parents often express concerns about phenomena that are in fact within the normal range.

- Minor posseting (spitting up) in a healthy, well-grown infant. Almost all infants have at least occasional posseting after feeds. If minor,

A case history

A mother at a well-baby clinic reported that her 4-month-old baby had lost his appetite over the past 24–48 hours. The baby was somewhat drowsy and the mother volunteered that he had vomited twice that day. She was reassured that it was too soon for concern about the baby's feeding and things would probably settle down. The next morning, she found her baby collapsed, unresponsive and grey. Despite the urgent efforts of the pediatric team in hospital, the baby died of meningitis.

this is not an indication for milk-switching, dietary manipulation, addition of milk thickeners or investigation for allergy. It usually ceases soon after the infant assumes the vertical posture and begins to walk. Reassurance is all that is needed.

- Infant crying or colic is very common in the first 3 months. While some practical suggestions may prove effective (see Chapter 8, page 68), it is often helpful to reassure the parents that there is no underlying disease process.
- Initial refusal of certain specific foods or even food groups: for infants who have only tasted milk, there may be a period of acclimatization to new tastes and textures. This is not a medical problem. Parents should continue to offer a variety of age-appropriate foods even if the infant initially refuses them.

Who should deal with this problem? Feeding problems may present initially to nurses, health visitors, breast feeding consultants, etc. Referral to a medical practitioner is generally indicated when:

- the baby is unwell
- there is impairment of growth or nutritional status
- there are abnormal clinical signs.

What action is needed? One or more of the following actions are needed in the management of a feeding problem:

- reassurance (if the 'problem' is not abnormal)
- parental education (e.g. if incorrect practice is identified; see Table 9.8, page 90)
- parental supervision and assistance (for many practical feeding problems)
- clinical examination of the baby (in the case of a sick child or growth failure)
- medical treatment of baby or mother (e.g. for a breast abscess)
- special investigations (if an underlying disorder is suspected)
- hospital referral – sometimes urgent (for acute illness presenting as a feeding disorder).

Is follow-up needed? Feeding is an important aspect of infant care that causes considerable uncertainty for parents and often raises continuing medical or social concerns for health professionals. Follow-up is often needed for the following reasons.

- Parents may not be adequately reassured in one session.
- Advice or education is often not absorbed in one session.
- Feeding problems may not resolve quickly and may require continuing management.
- Feeding problems can be a manifestation of inadequate, inappropriate or even neglectful parental care. When this is suspected, supervision or continued observation is needed.

Specific feeding problems

Some feeding-related problems are discussed in other chapters. Below, selected problems are considered according to the classification in the opening paragraph of this chapter.

Underlying illness presenting as a feeding problem. Anorexia, poor feeding and vomiting are non-specific symptoms that commonly occur under many circumstances in infants and young children. A primary role of the healthcare provider is to determine when these symptoms are manifestations of more serious diseases that need medical attention and will generally require specialist referral (Table 9.2).

Problems with the mechanics of feeding can be technical, functional or structural in origin.

Technical feeding difficulties are common and can reflect maternal inexperience. Breastfed babies may be unable to latch onto the breast or may clamp onto the nipple (which can traumatize it) as a result of suboptimal positioning of the baby on the breast. Appropriate positions for the breastfed infant are shown in Figure 9.1, and signs of good attachment at the breast are listed in Table 9.3.

Premature infants may have difficulty feeding for medical and neurodevelopmental reasons, but they may also have temporary, simple technical feeding difficulties, because their mouth is smaller and cannot easily encompass the mother's nipple or a regular feeding-bottle teat. Mothers may need help with attachment at the breast, and formula-fed babies may require specially designed feeding-bottle teats.

A functional problem with sucking, swallowing or coordination of feeding with breathing may be associated with a number of

TABLE 9.2

Underlying illnesses that may present as poor feeding or vomiting

- Viral or bacterial infections, including upper or lower respiratory tract infections, otitis media, meningitis, gastroenteritis, hepatitis, urinary tract or renal infections
- Structural abnormalities, e.g. congenital pyloric stenosis, gastroesophageal reflux, Hirschsprung's disease, intussusception, volvulus, posterior urethral valves
- Neurodevelopmental or neuromuscular disorders, including cerebral palsy and muscular dystrophy
- Inborn errors of metabolism, such as abnormalities of glycogen storage, vitamin D metabolism, and amino acid or lipid metabolism
- Tumors of the central nervous system, hematological system, kidney or adrenal glands

TABLE 9.3

Signs of good attachment to the breast*

- Lips turned outwards
- Nose and chin touch breast
- Nipple enclosed in the mouth 1–2 cm beyond its base
- Tongue visible if lower lip is pulled down

*After Hopkinson et al., in: Tsang RC et al., 1997

neurodevelopmental disturbances (Table 9.4). The problem may be minor and transient, or may reflect a more major condition, such as cerebral palsy. Feeding problems can also be the first, subtle manifestation of a neurodevelopmental disorder. Such problems may require specialist management (e.g. from a speech therapist); in more severe cases, nutritional support (e.g. gastrostomy feeding) may be required. Nevertheless, many babies that are difficult to feed will need to be managed in the community in collaboration with specialist teams (see below).

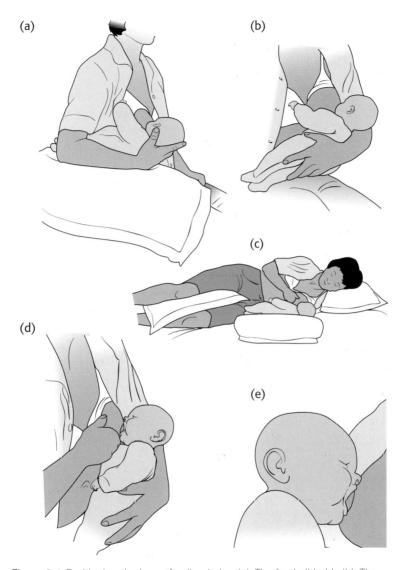

Figure 9.1 Positioning the breastfeeding baby. (a) The football hold. (b) The cradle hold. (c) After cesarean section, the mother may be more comfortable with a pillow placed between the legs to reduce the stress placed on the incision. (d) The mother's fingers must be positioned behind the areola so that they do not interfere with the infant's access. (e) Effective 'latch-on', with the lips turned outward, and the nose and chin touching the breast. Adapted with permission from Tsang RC et al., 1997.

TABLE 9.4

Neurodevelopmental causes of feeding problems

- Birth asphyxia and resulting cerebral palsy
- Adverse cerebral effects of illness (e.g. complications of prematurity, meningitis)
- Sequelae of head trauma (e.g. subdural hematoma)
- Cortical atrophy, microcephaly and hydrocephaly
- 'Minimal brain dysfunction'

Mechanical feeding difficulties can arise from structural, congenital abnormalities of the orofacial region (Table 9.5). While these require specialized treatment, some understanding of modern approaches is required by community-based health professionals (Table 9.6).

Problems apparently relating to the gut. Colic and constipation are discussed in Chapter 8 (page 68). Although minor posseting is normal (see page 83–4), more marked and sustained regurgitation or vomiting needs consideration. Vomiting in an ill baby should raise the question in the healthcare professional's mind of the possibility of significant underlying illness, often unrelated to the gut (see Table 9.2). Chronic regurgitation in an otherwise well infant, with or without evidence of

TABLE 9.5

Common congenital orofacial problems affecting feeding and swallowing

- Cleft lip and/or cleft palate
- Choanal atresia and stenosis
- Hypopharyngeal stenosis and webs
- Craniofacial syndromes with micrognathia (e.g. Pierre Robin, Crouzon, Treacher Collins, Goldenhar)
- Laryngeal stenosis, webs and paralysis, and laryngomalacia
- Tracheoesophageal fistula/esophageal atresia

TABLE 9.6

General approach to infants with dysfunctional swallowing

- Modification of volume and consistency of the formula
- Appropriate positioning of the head, neck and body during swallowing
- Modification of intraoral bolus placement
- Provision of jaw control and stabilization
- Valved bottle feeding
- Specialized teats
- Specialized techniques
  - swallowing exercises, including tongue resistance and range of motion and laryngeal adduction
  - modification of oral sensitivity
- Provision of an alternative to oral nutrition (e.g. nasogastric or enterostomy tube feeding)

impaired nutritional status, is a common feeding problem requiring diagnosis if possible and management advice. Evaluation of reflux commonly includes a barium swallow. Although this provides little useful physiological information such as the rate of gastric emptying, it is helpful in identifying infants with a large hiatal hernia, esophageal stricture, atypical pyloric stenosis, duodenal or gastric web or other anatomical cause of recurrent vomiting. The development of pediatric pH probes that can be placed in the esophagus for 24 hours or more, while still allowing the infant to function relatively normally, has facilitated more accurate diagnosis of gastroesophageal reflux disease (GERD) and monitoring of the response to pharmacological interventions. Evaluation of most babies with GERD reveals no definable anatomical, metabolic, infectious or neurological etiology, but a number of management strategies are available (Table 9.7).

Problems due to inappropriate feeding practices. Inappropriate feeding practices due to inexperience, lack of education or a parental 'philosophy' are common (Table 9.8). However, since many recommendations are not strictly evidence-based, minor deviation from

TABLE 9.7

Management of gastroesophageal reflux disease

Posture

- Head elevated to prone position after feeding (in a harness)

Drugs

- H_2-blockers to reduce the amount of acid in gastric contents and thus decrease esophagitis, and prokinetic drugs to decrease gastric emptying time and increase lower esophageal sphincter pressure

Surgery

- If necessary, to tighten the lower esophageal sphincter and prevent the reflux of gastric contents into the esophagus

Feeding

- Thickened feeds on their own are not effective for reflux, though this intervention seems worthwhile because it has been shown to decrease the number of episodes of vomiting, the time spent crying and the time spent awake

TABLE 9.8

Inappropriate feeding practices

- Failure to follow instructions for mixing formulas, resulting in feeds that are too dilute or too concentrated
- Use of unmodified cows' milk prior to recommended age
- Use of fat-reduced cows' milk (skimmed, 1%- or 2%-fat milk)
- Introduction of puréed foods prior to recommended time
- Excessive use of table salt in home-prepared puréed foods
- Use of 'empty' fast foods (e.g. fizzy drinks, candy, crisps)
- Excessive ingestion of fruit juices
- Use of foods that may cause choking because of their size or shape (e.g. nuts, raw carrots)
- Allowing a child to feed independently without adult supervision

the rules (e.g. introduction of tastes of weaning foods at 3 months) may be acceptable. Nevertheless, vigilance is required to detect more major deviations, which can be frankly unsafe (see also Chapter 8, page 68), or can result in overall undernutrition, specific nutritional insufficiencies or overnutrition.

Problems with feeding behavior and appetite. Impaired appetite and deranged feeding behavior can occur in many medical conditions. Two feeding issues are, however, common.

Food refusal and babies that are difficult to feed. Food refusal can range from mild (e.g. 'pickiness' or refusal to progress from liquids to new textures) to severe (total food refusal). Etiology is complex and it may be secondary to identifiable causes, such as the pain and discomfort associated with GERD and esophagitis, or forced feeding. Infants who have had traumatic oral experiences may learn to associate oral stimulation, including swallowing, with distress, fear, discomfort or pain, and are at risk of developing a conditioned or learned aversion to eating or drinking. The aversion might be due to a prior incident of choking or gagging on food or medicine. An estimated 40% of infants traumatized by medical, surgical or intrusive diagnostic procedures involving the esophagus may develop swallowing or feeding problems. Infants born prematurely are particularly at risk, because of traumatic procedures to the pharynx. Infants with severe food refusal may cry, gag or choke even at the mere sight of a bottle or food, refuse to have anything touch their lips or inserted in their mouth, refuse to chew or swallow, and often lack awareness of hunger. They may only accept a bottle when they are falling asleep. Such problems may be made worse by parental anxiety and inexperience.

These infants and indeed many others who are difficult to feed for a variety of reasons may respond to a structured approach to changing their feeding behavior (Table 9.9), which is based on the rationale that such infants must establish regular 'hunger–satiety' cycles. The practical implication of this principle is that infants and toddlers are more likely to be compliant with feeding if they are hungry and thirsty. This justifies a structured feeding schedule with meals limited to a maximum of 30 minutes and without snacks between meals. When children learn

TABLE 9.9

A structured approach to changing difficult feeding behavior

- Provide a structured mealtime schedule; for example, feed every 4 hours
- Offer small portions of food and give praise for eating the amount provided. Gradually increase the amount of food required to receive praise
- No food (snacks) provided between scheduled meals
- No drinks, with the exception of water, for up to 2 hours before the next meal
- Food should not be given as a present or reward
- Feed the baby in a quiet place with few distractions (no television or toys)
- The feeder should have a calm, positive attitude at mealtimes
- The baby should be positioned comfortably in a developmentally appropriate seat (i.e. a highchair if able to sit independently)
- A limited number of feeders (ideally one person) should feed the baby

Additional advice for managing toddlers

- Do not allow grazing
- Following a toddler around the home with food is inappropriate
- Meals should be time-limited (e.g. 30 minutes) and food removed after 10–15 minutes if the toddler seems to play with the food without eating
- The meal should be terminated if the child throws food in anger
- When mealtime is over, plates should be removed regardless of whether the child has finished – uneaten food should be removed without lectures or condemnation for not eating

to associate feeding with feelings of fullness and satiety, then feedings 'reinforce' and motivate appropriate feeding behavior.

Obesity. The sharp rise in obesity in the West has refocused interest on its early-life origins. However, infancy is often considered too young for intervention, especially as most overweight infants do not become overweight adults. Manipulation of milk feeding (e.g. fewer or shorter breastfeeds) to reduce body weight gain is certainly not recommended, and neither are the dietary strategies used for weight control in adults (i.e. dieting, reduced fat intake, use of low-fat milk or high fiber intake). Nevertheless, some health professionals find frank obesity in infancy hard to ignore. In such a case, the following suggestions may be helpful.

- Take a good feeding history.
- If inappropriate feeding practices that promote excessive intake are identified (e.g. incorrect formula reconstitution, use of weaning foods too early), education is required.
- Counsel parents on appropriate food choices, mealtimes and portion sizes if there is substantial deviation from the norm.
- Discuss excessive use of food as a reward.
- If the infant belongs to a family in which all members are overweight, the prognosis for the infant depends on the motivation of the whole family to change and accept advice.

Maternal problems affecting infant feeding. Contraindications to breastfeeding and drugs in breast milk are discussed in Chapter 4 (page 35). There are four common problems of the breast that affect infant feeding:

- breast engorgement
- sore nipples
- inverted nipples
- breast infection (mastitis).

Failure to attend to these problems quickly can result in impaired milk flow and therefore nutritional insufficiency in the infant.

Breast engorgement. Unrelieved breast engorgement is the greatest single physical cause of unsuccessful breastfeeding. Significant breast engorgement is common, with an incidence of 20% in primiparous mothers. The swelling makes infant attachment difficult; swelling of the nipple and areola increases the likelihood of nipple trauma and soreness; and engorgement reduces milk flow and, eventually, milk production. All these factors can impair infant nutrition. A number of measures can help to relieve the problem.

- Correct positioning of the baby is critical, and the baby must clamp on well beyond the nipple (see Figure 9.1 and Table 9.3).
- Expressing some milk manually or mechanically before feeding will facilitate attachment.

- While cupping the breast in the 'C' hold (thumb on top of breast, fingers below), and with fingers and thumb well behind the areola, the mother can compress the breast gently to shape the nipple and areola so that it is easier for the infant to attach.
- A good comfortable breast pump should be used to empty the breast if it is still engorged after feeding. Pumping will encourage milk flow, which is important in relieving the condition.

Sore nipples. Nipple pain that is sufficiently severe to lead to a dread of breastfeeding is experienced by 13% of new mothers (Neifert, 1998), yet it is a treatable condition. Untreated, sore nipples can lead to cessation of breastfeeding, impaired mother–infant interaction, poor milk flow and reduced infant growth. Mothers can be advised to take the following steps to reduce soreness.

- Ensure correct attachment with the mouth clamped well past the nipple (see Figure 9.1 and Table 9.3).
- Start feeding on the less sore nipple to establish flow.
- Give more frequent, shorter feeds.
- Keep the skin of the nipple dry after feeding.
- Cover cracks in the skin with lanolin-based ointment.
- Wear breast shells to protect nipples between nursing.
- Pump off excess milk if pain is severe.
- Use expressed milk for a while if the nipple is bleeding significantly. (Remember that blood in infant stools can be maternal in origin, and the hospital laboratory can test for this.)

Soreness may be due to yeast infection, in which case both mother and baby should be treated.

Inverted nipples. Flat or inverted nipples, which can affect breastfeeding, are seen in 10% of mothers. Social embarrassment leads some women to have plastic surgery that destroys subsequent breast function. A number of measures can help the problem.

- Hoffman's exercises, which involve regular manual manipulation to evert the nipple, or wearing a breast shield during pregnancy are common, especially the latter, but neither method has proven efficacy in clinical studies.
- Use of a breast pump to evert the nipple before feeding is helpful.

- A simple thimble-like device covering the nipple (the 'Nipplette') is connected to a syringe, and controlled suction is applied. This technique can correct the problem permanently after 2–3 months.

Breast infection (mastitis) occurs in 10% of nursing mothers and is caused by: poor breast emptying (insufficient infant feeding); blocked milk duct; and entry of organisms via a cracked nipple. Mastitis usually presents with breast pain, soreness, redness and flu-like symptoms.

Mothers should continue to breastfeed, as this encourages milk flow and drainage, and the organisms are likely to have come from the infant in any case. Antibiotics should be given, which will be secreted into the breast milk. A good fluid intake should be maintained and analgesia given as required. Breastfeeding from the affected breast should be stopped temporarily if there is frank pus in the milk, and the milk should be expressed.

Failure to thrive at the breast. Despite the discomfort this issue engenders in some breastfeeding advocates, insufficient breast-milk intake is not uncommon and, if unrecognized, can lead to poor growth and, eventually, frank malnutrition and dehydration.

According to Neifert, primary lactation failure occurs in only 2–5% of breastfeeding mothers, and may be associated with abnormalities of breast development, prior surgery, endocrine disorders, radiation damage, chronic maternal illness or malnutrition. Secondary causes of insufficient milk intake by the infant are, however, more common. The most common cause is unrelieved breast engorgement; other causes include inadequate breast emptying (e.g. infrequent nursing, poor positioning of the infant), separation of mother and infant, maternal illness, some drugs and maternal undernutrition. If insufficient breast-milk intake is suspected, the following steps should be taken.

- The diagnosis of failure to thrive should be verified in terms of poor growth and poor weight for height (Chapter 3, page 23), or excessive postnatal weight loss (sustained loss of > 10% of birthweight for ≥ 4 days).
- It must not be assumed that failure to thrive is a breastfeeding problem; the infant should be examined for other disorders.

- A good history should be taken and breastfeeding observed in order to identify the likely cause of the problem; primary failure of lactation is usually intractable, but secondary milk insufficiency is often treatable.

Steps to increase the milk supply include the following.

- Manage the underlying problem (e.g. engorgement).
- Advise more frequent and/or longer feeds.
- Ensure good feeding technique (see Figure 9.1 and Table 9.3).
- Ensure adequate maternal hydration.
- Advise use of a milk pump to further encourage milk flow.
- Consider metoclopramide, 10 mg three times daily, to increase milk flow; however, this is not always effective and can lead to side-effects (e.g. headache, sedation, depression).

The primary objective, however, is to ensure adequate infant nutrition, and supplementary feeding (generally infant formula) may be required, if possible accompanied by continuation of breastfeeding. This is an area for sensitive and skilled management in keen breastfeeders.

TABLE 9.10

Professional experience needed by those giving advice on feeding

- See breastfeeding in action (many younger doctors have never seen breastfeeding)
- Reconstitute infant formula from powder or concentrate (under supervision), using manufacturer's instructions
- Visit a supermarket to examine the range of products available for weaning healthy infants and study the product information closely
- Personally administer a formula feed
- Feed solid foods to a young infant
- Feed babies who are difficult to feed (e.g. those with mechanical or neurological feeding problems)
- See common problems with the breast (e.g. engorgement, sore or cracked nipples, mastitis)
- Practice taking a feeding history

Professional training and experience

Feeding and nutrition, though interrelated, are not the same, and the professional skills required to manage them are quite different. Expertise in nutritional problems is more common than that in feeding problems, which is an area that requires clinical acumen, experience and patience.

Medical training may inadequately equip professionals to give practical advice on simple infant feeding problems. Medical educators need to encourage professionals-in-training to attain the basic practical experience (Table 9.10) they need in order to advise mothers.

This book outlines a standard of practice for infant nutrition – a practice justified largely on the basis of short-term studies. However, the most robust way of justifying nutritional practice is on the basis of formal outcome trials, notably trials that explore the effects of early nutrition on long-term health and development.

Nutritional programming

Extensive animal data now demonstrate the potential lifetime, broad-based programming effects of early nutrition on blood pressure, obesity, diabetic tendency, atherosclerosis, learning behavior and longevity. The important issue has been whether such programming occurs in humans.

In recent studies on premature babies, as little as 4 weeks of randomized dietary manipulation has had major long-term effects. Feeding these infants on a special nutrient-enriched preterm infant formula (designed to meet their calculated increased nutritional needs for somatic and brain growth) compared with a standard formula resulted in a 12-point increase in verbal IQ in boys at 7.5–8 years of follow-up. This is likely to be permanent. Optimal early nutrition also appears important for long-term bone health. In another parallel intervention study, preterm infants randomly assigned to banked, donor breast milk in the early weeks had lower blood pressure and LDL cholesterol 13–16 years later than those assigned a nutrient-enriched formula. In a further study, those fed on the most nutrient-enriched diets showed evidence of greater insulin resistance in adolescence.

Evidence is now accumulating that the later health of healthy full-term infants is also influenced by their early nutrition. These data demonstrate the unexpected sensitivity of infants to their nutritional environment during critical periods of development. Such findings must be seen alongside numerous observational studies in humans linking possible early markers of nutrition (size and growth in early life) with disease in later life, including high blood pressure, diabetes, obesity and death from ischemic heart disease.

These data have major future public health and biological implications. The next frontier of research into infant nutrition will be to establish experimentally those aspects of early nutrition that have significance for future health. We cannot afford to have preformed views. For example, should we worry about infants on the 98th centile for weight at 1 year in terms of later obesity risk, when it has been shown in over 5000 males that the heavier an infant is at 1 year the *lower* the risk of death from ischemic heart disease in the sixth and seventh decades of life?

The relationship between early nutrition and later outcome may prove complex. Primates assigned to breastfeeding appear to be programmed to be conservative with cholesterol, which would be 'adaptive' in their natural habitat. But if these breastfed animals are then placed unphysiologically on a Western-style diet that is rich in saturated fats, they show adverse long-term changes in the lipid pattern (raised LDL and lowered HDL cholesterol, and increased cholesterol absorption); and at post mortem, more atherosclerosis than those fed infant formula. If such interactions between infant nutrition and subsequent diet turn out to be applicable to humans (two published Western studies indicate prolonged breastfeeding is associated with later ischemic heart disease in males, or impaired vascular distensibility at age 20–30 years), we may need to ensure that initial milk feeding leads on to the most appropriate transitional and childhood foods. Until now, planning of nutritional advice in childhood has not been based on such considerations.

Small-for-gestational-age (SGA) full term infants will be an important target group. They are at risk for ischemic heart disease and its antecedents. Recently, SGA infants have been shown (unpublished) to be amenable to short-term nutritional 'rescue' by increasing the plane of their nutrition during a window in early infancy. The enhancing effects on observed growth appear to persist into early childhood, beyond the period of dietary randomization. Will such nutritional rescue reprogram these infants to reduce their otherwise increased risk of diabetes, hypertension and atherosclerotic disease? Or will early growth promotion make matters even worse, bearing in mind that in species as diverse as butterflies, frogs, salmon, rats and baboons rapid early growth may adversely affect long-term health or longevity?

Investigative tools

Clearly, infants randomly assigned to their early diet cannot be practically followed up for life. Tools are being developed to explore, non-invasively, whether infant nutrition has had adverse or beneficial programming effects. For example, vascular ultrasound can now be used to test for nitric-oxide-mediated endothelial dysfunction in children as the first indicator of atherosclerotic disease. Already, 9- to 11-year-old schoolchildren have been shown to have increased vascular dysfunction if they are small in early life. Sophisticated magnetic resonance imaging (MRI) studies of the brain are now being used to demonstrate the effects of early nutrition on the structure of the brain in relation to function in adolescence and early adult life.

Mechanisms

Given the broad human and animal evidence for nutritional programming, an understanding of the fundamental biological mechanisms involved is required. How, for example, is the 'memory' of an early nutritional experience retained in the body through many cell generations to be expressed in later life? Proposed mechanisms include adaptive effects on gene expression, clonal selection of cell types 'adapted' to the early nutritional environment, and differential cell proliferation at an early stage resulting in changes in the proportion of cell types in tissues. Understanding such fundamental processes may ultimately enable us to use nutrients in an intelligent and targeted way to affect the 'operating system' of our genome to influence future health.

Overview

The implication is that we can no longer consider nutrition simply in terms of meeting nutritional needs. We must consider the biological effects of nutrition, which can have important effects on the genome, on developmental biology, and on short- and long-term health. Given the hitherto unexpected importance of early nutrition, there is now a new onus on health professionals to focus on clinical nutritional care and for researchers to undertake formal long-term efficacy and safety studies to underpin developments in practice. Current evidence suggests early nutrition will become a major public health focus in the 21st century.

Useful addresses

Child Growth Foundation
2 Mayfield Avenue
London W4 1PW
Tel: 020 8995 0257
Fax: 020 8995 9075
cgflondon@aol.com
www.heightmatters.org.uk

Child Growth Foundation growth charts are available from:
Harlow Printing
Maxwell St
South Shields NE33 4PU (UK)
Tel: 0191 455 4286
Fax: 0191 427 0195
sales@harlowprinting.co.uk

Canadian Paediatric Society
www.cps.ca

American Academy of Pediatrics
PO Box 927
141 Northwest Point Boulevard
Elk Grove Village
Illinois 60007-1098
www.aap.org

British Dietetic Association
www.bda.uk.com

UK Food Standards Agency
www.foodstandards.gov.uk

American Dietetic Association
www.eatright.org

US Food and Nutrition Board
(RDAs)
www.nationalacademies.org/iom/iomhome.nsf/pages/food+and+nutrition+board

US Department of Agriculture
www.usda.gov/cnpp

US Food and Nutrition
Information Center
www.nal.usda.gov/fnic

Key references and further reading

American Academy of Pediatrics, ed. *Pediatric Nutrition Handbook*. 4th edn. Elk Grove Village: AAP, 1999.

Fomon SJ. *Nutrition of Normal Infants*. St Louis: Mosby–Year Book, 1993.

Lucas A. Programming by early nutrition: an experimental approach. *J Nutr* 1998;128(2 suppl):401–6S.

Lucas A, Fewtrell M. Nutritional physiology. Part I: dietary requirements of full- and preterm infants. Part II: Feeding the full-term infant. In: Rennie JM, Robertson NRC, eds. *Textbook of Neonatology*. 3rd edn. London: Churchill Livingstone, 1999: part 1, 305–48.

Neifert M. *Dr Mom's Guide to Breastfeeding*. New York: Plume, 1998.

Roberts SB, Heyman MB, Tracy L. *Feeding Your Child for Lifelong Health*. New York: Bantam, 1999.

Subcommittee on the tenth edition of the RDAs. *Recommended Dietary Allowances*. 10th edn. Washington DC: Food and Nutrition Board, Commission on Life Sciences, National Research Council, National Academy Press, 1989.

Standing Committee on the Scientific Evaluation of Dietary Reference Intakes. *Dietary reference intakes for calcium, phosphorus, magnesium, vitamin D and fluoride*. Washington DC: Food and Nutrition Board, Institute of Medicine, National Academy Press, 1989.

Standing Committee on the Scientific Evaluation of Dietary Reference Intakes. *Dietary reference intakes for vitamin A, vitamin K, arsenic, boron, chromium, copper, iodine, iron, manganese, molybdenum, nickel, silicon, vanadium, and zinc*. Food and Nutrition Board, Institute of Medicine, National Academy Press, Washington DC, 2000. (SZ is a contributing author.)

Tsang RC, Uuay R, Lucas A, Zlotkin SH, eds. *Nutritional Needs of the Preterm Infant: Scientific Basis and Practical Guidelines*. New York: Williams & Wilkins, 1993.

Tsang RC, Zlotkin SH, Nichols BL, Hansen JW, eds. *Nutrition During Infancy – Principles and Practice*. Cincinnati, Ohio: Digital Education Publishing, 1997.

Wells JCK, Cole TJ, Davies PSW. Total energy expenditure and body composition in early infancy. *Arch Dis Child* 1996;75:423–6.

Zeiger RS. Food allergen avoidance in the prevention of food allergy in infants and children. *Pediatrics* 2003;11:1662–71.

Index